ABC of
Evidence-Based Healthcare

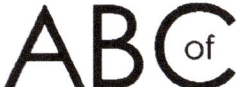

Evidence-Based Healthcare

Edited by

John Frain

Division of Medical Sciences and Graduate Entry Medicine
University of Nottingham
Nottingham, UK

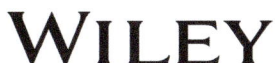

Registered Office(s)

John Wiley & Sons, Inc., 111 River Street, Hoboken, NJ 07030, USA

John Wiley & Sons Ltd, New Era House, 8 Oldlands Way, Bognor Regis, West Sussex, PO22 9NQ, UK

For details of our global editorial offices, customer services, and more information about Wiley products visit us at www.wiley.com.

The manufacturer's authorized representative according to the EU General Product Safety Regulation is Wiley-VCH GmbH, Boschstr. 12, 69469 Weinheim, Germany, e-mail: Product_Safety@wiley.com.

Wiley also publishes its books in a variety of electronic formats and by print-on-demand. Some content that appears in standard print versions of this book may not be available in other formats.

Library of Congress Cataloging-in-Publication Data Applied for:

Paperback ISBN: 9781394219315

Cover Design: Wiley

Cover Images: © Wightman JM. Radial Pulse Quality as a Diagnostic Testin Tactical Combat Casualty Care. Mil Med. 2020 Dec 30;185(11-12):484-486.doi: 10.1093/milmed/usaa199. PMID: 32779710. CC BY 4.0, © The Good Brigade/Getty Images

Set in 9.25/12pt Minion by Straive, Pondicherry, India

Printed in Singapore

M WEP343713 100225

Contents

List of Contributors

John Frain
Division of Medical Sciences and Graduate Entry Medicine
University of Nottingham, Nottingham, UK

Alistair Hewins
Final Year Graduate Entry Medical Student, University of Nottingham
Nottingham, UK

Raj Himatshih Babla
Division of Medical Sciences and Graduate Entry Medicine
University of Nottingham, Nottingham, UK
Clinical Implementation Lead, Stoneygate Centre for Empathic Healthcare
University of Leicester, Leicester, UK

Preface

I am writing this book not as a researcher but as an end user of evidence-based healthcare. What does this mean? It means I am a frontline clinician, in primary care, working to provide patients with care and management according to the best available evidence, helping them to interpret what they have seen, most commonly now, online but also in newspapers, on TV or simply by word of mouth from family and friends. I need to know how to retrieve and interpret evidence quickly and accurately. I need evidence to collaborate with my patients and to share decision-making with them in line with their own preferences and values. Practising in primary care is often about the management of uncertainty – not only the patient's but also mine and my team's. The prospect of making our work more evidence-based to assist our clinical judgement is certainly an attractive one. Healthcare is a team-based activity, and the well-being of patients is dependent on the well-being of the staff. During the recent Covid-19 pandemic, my practice continued to see our patients face-to-face whenever necessary. In a previously unknown and rapidly evolving situation, the availability of high-quality evidence was essential in keeping our patients and staff safe.

The full implementation of evidence in healthcare is not a fixed endpoint nor even a destination to which we are yet close. Humankind has always sought to interpret the causes of disease and the benefits of available treatments. Though the quality of evidence for healthcare has improved immeasurably over the past 30 years, there remain challenges. These involve greater implementation of evidence into healthcare policy, everyday practice and the lives of patients, staff and healthcare providers. Amazingly, the 'evidence cart' can now be held in the hand and stored in the pocket. The technological revolution of the information age enables rapid retrieval of evidence to aid bedside decision-making with just a few clicks. Yet not all available evidence is published, not every trial is well conducted and not every healthcare professional and policymaker is skilled in the appraisal of evidence. Still too often, historically underserved and marginalised individuals and communities remain outside the remit of mainstream research, reinforcing their often-poorer health outcomes. This must change, and we have the tools to do this.

As an educator, I am aware of the great volume of knowledge and assessment with which healthcare students must contend. Evidence-based healthcare can seem abstract and lacking relevance if it is only placed alongside other learning themes rather than embedded across the whole curriculum, informing the choice of what is to be taught to future healthcare professionals. Students need to become familiar with the skills and the benefits of evidence-based healthcare right from the beginning of their training rather than seeing it as an 'add-on' for a later date.

It is not within the scope of this book to cover everything in evidence-based healthcare. I have tried to address the important domains across the skill set as well as to provoke thought for the reader of implementation and future challenges. Underpinning this, I have added details of suitable further resources readers may also wish to review.

Finally, I would like to thank everyone who has contributed to this book and to Wiley who have supported it from concept to publication. I hope it is useful and helps to provide the reader with an overview of this important topic in healthcare and provides direction to other resources and further study.

John Frain
August 2024

CHAPTER 1

What Is Evidence-Based Healthcare?

John Frain

Division of Medical Sciences and Graduate Entry Medicine, University of Nottingham, Nottingham, UK

OVERVIEW

- Evidence is the available information or facts which indicate whether a belief or proposition is true.
- Evidence in healthcare is linked to quality, patient safety and improved clinical outcomes.
- The concept of justifying practice through the use of evidence can be found from the earliest times.
- Modern evidence-based practice has its roots in the development of critical appraisal and modern research methods.
- The ethical dimension is essential in determining the quality and application of evidence.

Introduction

On explaining to a fellow new student on another university course that I was studying evidence-based healthcare and how to bring evidence into our clinical practice, the alarmed response I received was, 'You mean healthcare isn't already evidence-based?' It seems obvious that something as important as healthcare should proceed only on the basis of the evidence, given the possible consequences of poor practice. The answer to my colleague's concern is, of course, both 'Yes, it is' and 'No, it isn't or rather 'There is evidence, but it could be better, both in terms of the knowledge and how the knowledge is applied to patient care'. It is always this tension between where practice is now and where it could be in the future, which should motivate both scientists and clinicians to always develop the scope of evidence further in our practice.

Evidence is not only static but also dynamic in the sense our depth of understanding should always be evolving. An example is finger clubbing, first described by Hippocrates in a patient with empyema in the sixth century BCE. Our understanding of clubbing is different from 2500 years ago (Box 1.1).

Therefore, observation is crucial in healthcare because it raises curiosity about the origin of the data, and in this case a physical sign clinicians see in their patients. Hippocrates' initial observation of a patient's fingers and his curiosity about a relationship (coincidence, association or causation?) with their empyema has evolved into an evidence-based physical sign which remains important in physical diagnosis. These clinical questions are vital in clinical reasoning and decision-making about a patient's management. They divide into questions about general knowledge of a condition, disease or process (background questions) and specific questions to facilitate clinical decision about the patient in front of us (foreground questions) (Chapter 2) (Box 1.2).

The volume of medical knowledge and belief has evolved immensely. Currently, Medline is adding over a million new records to its database every year. Hippocrates alone wrote around 60 treatises (the *Hippocratic Corpus*) describing theories of disease, ethical dimensions and approaches to observation and physical examination. Now every busy clinician appreciates the need to access high-quality information quickly and efficiently for the immediate benefit of patients. The need to summarise evidence and manage changing medical knowledge has been recognised since the seventeenth century with the publication of an abstracting journal in 1682 and the first medical journal in England, *Medicina Curiosa*, in 1684 (1). The development of indexing, databases and computerisation in the twentieth century has provided the automated databases and evidence retrieval we enjoy now, particularly in the last 30 years. These have facilitated an explosion in the opportunities for a more systematic and rigorous consideration of scientific evidence, which informs clinical practice today (Chapter 3). Many of us will remember the previous challenges of retrieving references for our student essays from the hefty volumes of the *Index Medicus*, followed by a search of the dusty shelves of a medical library stack room.

Comparing similar groups whose baseline characteristics are similar is particularly important in evaluating a new intervention and is the basis of the randomised controlled trial (RCT). Again, the concept has a long history, with the poet Francisco Petrarch proposing in the fourteenth century that the effects of then-current treatments for conditions in one group be compared with a similar group of patients in which the natural history of the condition was allowed to proceed unchecked. A famous example is James Lind's intervention in sailors with scurvy in 1747 (Box 1.3). The first recognised RCT is of the use of streptomycin in the treatment of pulmonary tuberculosis (2). Given the inherent variability of biological systems both individually and in populations, the precise comparison of groups required in accurately evaluating the effectiveness of interventions

---

ABC of Evidence-Based Healthcare, First Edition. Edited by John Frain.
© 2025 John Frain. Published 2025 by John Wiley & Sons Ltd.

Box 1.1 **Understanding the clinical significance of finger clubbing 'Hippocratic fingers'**

Clubbing is characterised by a bulbous swelling of the terminal phalanges of the fingers. It was described first by Hippocrates, who observed it in a patient with empyema. Later it was found to be associated with many conditions, including bronchiectasis, lung cancer, liver cirrhosis, cyanotic congenital heart disease and infective endocarditis. In 1976, South African cardiologist Leo Shamroth observed in his own clubbed fingers an obliteration of the diamond-shaped spaced normally seen when the dorsal surface of the nails are brought into contact with one another (Shamroth's sign). A study in *JAMA* in 2010 found inter-examiner agreement using Shamroth's sign on the presence of clubbing to give *kappa* values of 0.3–0.9 and concluded its use reasonable in the identification of clubbing. Clubbing is present in 1% of patients admitted acutely to acute medical wards and is associated with serious disease in 40% of these patients.

Source: Pallarés-Sanmartín et al. (20), Vandemergel and Renneboog (21).

Box 1.2 **Examples of background and foreground questions**

Background questions identify knowledge and understanding of disease processes or clinical conditions. They are often broad in scope and may be answerable from textbooks, general online sources and review articles. They may help information decision-making about a foreground question and a particular patient but are not the answers in themselves about what is appropriate for a particular patient.

Example – What is the pathophysiology and prognosis of acute otitis media in children under two years?

Foreground questions require knowledge to assist decision-making. They may involve a comparison of treatment options, including intervention. Answers to foreground questions require synthesis of primary studies and a comprehensive literature search. These may be used to produce an evidence summary or systematic review.

Example – Will prescribing oral antibiotics to my 18-month-old patient with acute otitis media improve or have any effect on their long-term prognosis?

has led to the development of medical statistics to describe these effects accurately (Chapter 6).

Healthcare before evidence-based healthcare

Evidence existed before the 1990s, and anyone practising in that era knows clinicians both aspired to and did practise scientifically for the benefit of patients. What happened in 1992 and afterwards happened because of what came before, as well as the development of innovative technology and the inspirational leadership of individuals and academic departments in articulating a new vision for the evaluation and application of evidence in healthcare. First is the improvement in the evaluation of interventions and treatments. This has been

Box 1.3 **James Lind and comparison of similar groups in the treatment of scurvy**

Scurvy results from a lack of vitamin D. It was particularly prevalent in the Royal Navy in the eighteenth century. Provision of citrus fruits to Dutch sailors suggested a reduction in the disease. In 1747, James Lind, a Royal Navy surgeon, selected 12 sailors with scurvy 'as similar as I could have them'. All sailors received the same diet. The sailors were divided into groups of two. Two were given a quart of cider each day, two took vitriol three times daily, two took two spoonfuls of vinegar daily, two were given seawater and two were given dietary supplements. The remaining two were each given two oranges and one lemon every day. 'The most sudden and visible effects were perceived from the use of oranges and lemons one being at the end of six days fit for duty and the other appointed to attend the rest of the sick'.

(Dr James Lind's Treatise on Scurvy, 1753)

Source: Adapted from Bhatt (19).

Table 1.1 A light-hearted perspective on alternatives to evidence-based medicine.

- Evidence-based medicine – relies on the randomised controlled trial and the systematic review
- Eminence-based medicine – the precedence of seniority of years in making the correct decision
- Vehemence-based medicine – the stridency with which one makes one's own beliefs known
- Eloquence-based medicine – the ability of ensuring one's views prevail given an ability to explain them beautifully
- Diffidence-based medicine – accepting the inevitability of the natural history of the patient's disease
- Nervousness-based medicine – practising with the aim of avoiding complaint or litigation

Source: Adapted from Straus et al. (3).

achieved through better study design, including registration of trials, protocols and promotion of reporting standards (Chapter 4). In addition, the promotion of critical appraisal skills, including in healthcare training programmes, has enabled practitioners to exercise greater reflection and discernment in how to apply evidence to their own patients (Chapters 7 and 8). Even though light-hearted in tone and certainly not advocated as viable alternatives, Isaacs and Fitzgerald's perspectives on evidence-based healthcare were written as a necessary counterpoint to the evidence-based approach and the issues raised by it. It is worth reflecting on Isaacs and Fitzgerald's thoughts on alternative methods of clinical decision-making (Table 1.1). In all things, there should always be a healthy scepticism, if only to encourage necessary questioning and debate to flourish.

The philosophy of evidence-based healthcare (4)

Healthcare is about diagnosis but at least as importantly about management including treatment and intervention. Historically, three approaches have been taken. Firstly, the impact of expertise

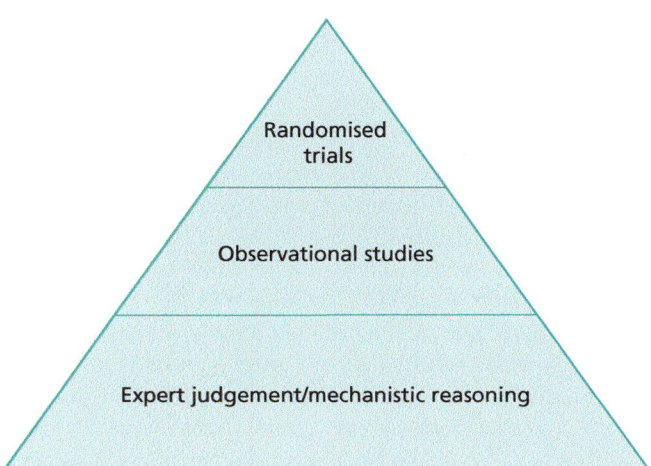

Figure 1.1 Simplified hierarchy of evidence (systematic review of all study types is assumed to be superior to single studies). *Source:* Howick (4)/John Wiley & Sons.

and experience allied to mechanistic reasoning ('In my experience, from the patients I have seen…'). There is also the approach that any treatment can only be deemed curative if the precise mechanism is known and understood. The final approach, advocated in evidence-based healthcare, is that the effects of a medical intervention are best evaluated by direct observation of the effects by comparing groups as similar as they can be – one which has received the intervention and one which has not. All the aforementioned constitute evidence, but a hierarchy of evidence exists (Figure 1.1) (4):

- Randomised trials (RCTs) or systematic reviews of many randomised trials offer stronger evidential support than observational studies.
- Comparative clinical studies in general (including both RCTs and observational studies) offer stronger evidential support than mechanistic reasoning from more basic sciences.
- Comparative clinical studies in general (including both RCTs and observational studies) offer stronger evidential support than expert clinical judgement.

The first decades of evidence-based healthcare have seen this approach become well established across clinical practice. At the same time, other themes have also emerged which were not initially considered (Chapter 9). For example, the perspectives of the patient and practitioner are both important in translating evidence into practice, and qualitative evaluation of these perspectives is also required. Moreover, clinical experience and expertise remain important, particularly in the realm of integrating policy, resources and shared decision-making with patients. Finally, though the robustness of study design and reporting has improved, historically marginalised and underserved populations remain underrepresented in research participation. This limits the wider application of evidence into practice.

The origins of the evidence-based healthcare movement

The 'Evidence-Based Medicine' movement was launched in the early 1990s by a group of epidemiologists at McMaster University, Hamilton, Canada. The aim was a new paradigm of medical practice. Proponents advocated greater reliance on published data

with evidence from clinical trials considered superior to mechanistic reasoning and clinical judgement (5). The concept of hierarchies of evidence developed during the 1970s (6). This culminated in 1981 with the publication of a series of articles in the *Canadian Medical Association Journal* on how to appraise the medical literature (7). While the principles of evidence-based medicine were quickly accepted into practice, nonetheless there was concern about restriction of clinical judgement, 'cookbook medicine' and use of evidence-based medicine by policymakers to implement cost-cutting measures. These concerns were rebutted by the authors in an excellent *BMJ* article published in 1996, which stated (8):

'Evidence based medicine is the conscientious, explicit, and judicious use of current best evidence in making care about the care of individual patients'.

Furthermore, the authors were clear that this meant integrating the best available evidence from systematic research with individual clinical expertise and that this increased expertise arises from effective and efficient diagnosis in combination with thoughtful identification and compassionate use of individual patients' predicaments, rights and preferences in decisions about their care. In the opinion of the authors, clinically relevant research may be from the basic sciences but especially from patient-centred research, including diagnostic accuracy, prognostic markers and the efficacy and safety of therapeutic, rehabilitative and preventive management (8). While well-conducted clinical trials and systematic reviews represent particularly high-quality research, this does not invalidate other well-designed studies if they are relevant and appropriate to the patient's presenting problem. This correlates all the areas from which clinical questions from both patients and practitioners are likely to arise and which reflect the domains of evidence-based healthcare:

- Aetiology/harm (causation)
- Prevention
- Diagnosis
- Therapy (treatment)
- Prognosis
- Meaning (patient's experiences)

Using evidence at the bedside

Healthcare is a high-pressure, time-limited activity which relies on the interaction and co-operation of all team members for the safety of the patient. This is facilitated by the availability of evidence. A feasibility study in 1995 at the University of Oxford, UK, concluded that making evidence available quickly to busy clinicians increased evidence-seeking and the incorporation of evidence into patient care decisions (9). An 'evidence cart' was taken on clinical rounds (Figure 1.2). On average, two to three questions arose for each patient. It took between 15 and 90 seconds to find relevant evidence (9). Evidence was found most quickly using a resource of pre-appraised topics, followed by use of *Best Evidence* with a Medline search taking the longest. Evidence changed management in one-third of patients (Table 1.2).

The development of tablets and handheld devices has overcome the practical challenges of a 'cart'. Clinicians are now used to retrieving

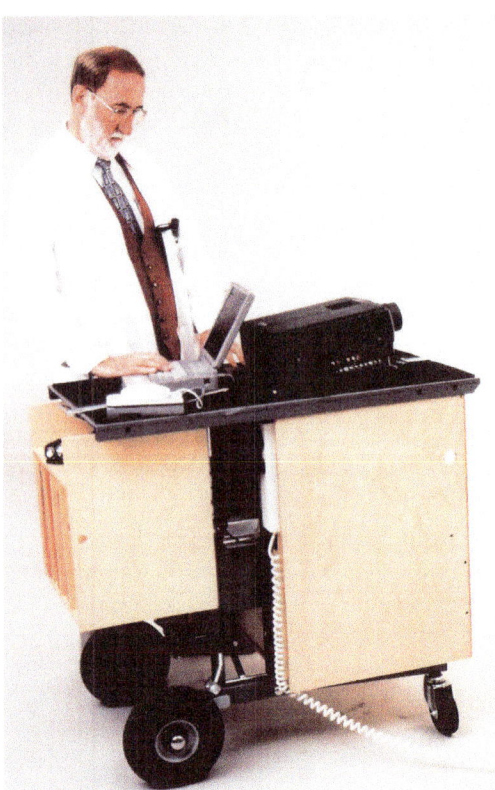

Figure 1.2 David Sacket demonstrating the evidence cart. *Source:* Straus et al. (10)/with permission of Sage Publications.

Table 1.2 Impact of the evidence cart.

- 81% – affected diagnosis and/or treatment
- 52% – confirmed current or tentative diagnostic or treatment plans
- 25% – led to new diagnostic skills, additional tests and new management decision
- 23% – corrected previous clinical skill, diagnostic test or treatment
- The perceived need for evidence was high, but search was done in only 12% of patients

Source: Adapted from Sackett and Straus (9).

evidence from their devices, even in front of patients. It is considered in the interests of patient safety and presents a cultural change from the perception the doctor must already know everything and be seen to already know everything. The development of pre-appraised sources and guidelines facilitates this, though time is still a limiting factor. Even so, evidence-based healthcare is not simply looking up evidence and what to do. Evidence must be assimilated and reasoned through even within the few seconds it takes to make a clinical decision. This approach needs to be embedded in training curricula – both undergraduate and postgraduate (Chapter 10). Use of evidence should permeate the whole of the clinical assessment and management pathways, including the history and examination. Teaching and learning evidence-based healthcare is not simply critical appraisal. It needs to be taught imaginatively to engage learners, and it should relate to their current experience. The content of healthcare courses should reflect the best evidence and how to apply it rather than simply where to find it. Learners should have the opportunity to apply evidence to patients they have encountered under supervision and receive feedback on their progress.

The achievements of evidence-based healthcare

Evidence-based healthcare has been forefront in the development of healthcare over the past 30 years. Its launch coincided with the growth of clinical guidelines. Guidelines have become influential in disseminating research evidence to frontline practitioners. The rigorous application of study design and reporting standards to medical research is essential in bringing structure and quality to the explosion of information and knowledge available via the internet. Ensuring treatments and interventions are applied only once they are rigorously and scientifically evaluated is essential in reducing patient harm and the overuse of technologies. The promotion of RCTs and systematic literature reviews (SLRs) has been both instrumental in focusing medical progress in interventions, treatments and devices firmly on an evidence base.

A particular achievement is the Cochrane Collaboration (Box 1.4). Founded in the United Kingdom and sponsored by the UK Department of Health, it has grown to an organisation of over 40 000 volunteers from over 190 countries responsible for producing over 400 systematic reviews each year on a wide range of medical treatments. Cochrane's members and supporters include researchers, health professionals, patients and carers. Worldwide 3.66 billion people have point-of-use access to the library (11). Over 7500 systematic reviews have been published by the Cochrane Library, where they are downloaded over 12.5 million times each year (Tables 1.3 and 1.4) (11).

Medical knowledge is more readily available to patients and non-clinicians. Healthcare practitioners are expected to share their knowledge in collaboration with patients in management. These conversations need to be evidence-based. Integrating evidence with clinical communication to share decision-making with patients is a recognised domain of clinical reasoning applicable in many areas of practice (12–14). Evidence-based practices consistently improve patient outcomes and returns on investment for healthcare providers (15).

Box 1.4 **The Cochrane database of systematic reviews**

The Cochrane Library is an international research network made up of several databases relating to biomedical research and associated economic analyses. The Cochrane Database of Systematic Reviews (CDSR) is an online repository of high-quality systematic reviews covering a wide range of topics. Cochrane reviews all follow guidelines for research methods relating to research question scope, systematically collecting evidence, assessing bias, statistical analysis and performing meta-analyses of amalgamated datasets. These guidelines are free to view online at https://training.cochrane.org/handbooks. The full texts of completed systematic reviews are freely available on the CDSR due to the Cochrane Library's commitment to open-access research. Protocols of completed and ongoing systematic reviews are also freely available and are a useful source for those wanting to better understand research methods for literature reviews.

Author: Alistair Hewins, Final Year Graduate Entry Medical Student, University of Nottingham, UK

Table 1.3 Types of review published by the Cochrane Library.

Intervention review	Assess the effectiveness/safety of a treatment, vaccine, device, preventative measure, procedure or policy
Diagnostic test accuracy review	Assess the accuracy of a test, device or scale to aid diagnosis
Prognosis review	Describe and predict the course of individuals with a disease or health condition
Qualitative evidence syntheses	Investigate perspectives and experiences of an intervention or health condition
Methodology reviews	Explore or validate how research is designed, conducted, reported or used
Overviews of reviews	Synthesise information from multiple systematic reviews on related research
Rapid reviews	Are systematic reviews accelerated through streamlining or omitting specific methods
Prototype reviews	Include other types of systematic review that do not yet have established standard methodology in Cochrane, such as scoping reviews, mixed-methods reviews, reviews of prevalence studies and realist reviews

Author: Alistair Hewins, Final Year Graduate Entry Medical Student, University of Nottingham, UK.

Table 1.4 Themes and examples of Cochrane library systematic reviews.

Themes	Published reviews	Example topics
Allergy and intolerance	63	Eczema Vaccinations Asthma
Cancer	833	Bone loss prevention Gene therapy Chemotherapy and biologic therapy Surgical management
Diagnosis	173	Triage/screening tools for spine injuries Measuring drug therapy adherence Imaging methods for diagnosis Novel tests for sepsis
Mental health	693	Antipsychotic effectiveness comparisons Risk assessments for schizophrenia Cognitive rehabilitation
Ear, nose and throat	218	Vestibular migraine management Virtual reality training for surgeons Management of acute otitis media
Gynaecology	382	Pain management in dysmenorrhoea Urinary incontinence management Surgical methods in hysterectomy
Public health	117	Implementing policies for diet, physical activity and tobacco use in schools Interventions for reducing social isolation in older people Fortification of foods to target malnutrition in the general population
Rheumatology	344	Nonmedical management of systemic lupus erythematosus Management of osteoporosis Pain management in rheumatoid arthritis

Author: Alistair Hewins, Final Year Graduate Entry Medical Student, University of Nottingham, UK.

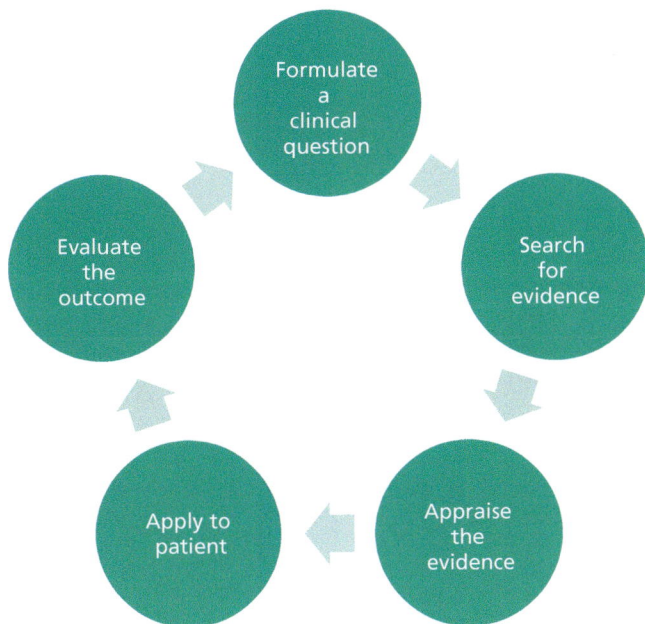

Figure 1.3 The five key steps of evidence-based healthcare.

The key steps of evidence-based healthcare

Whether researcher, frontline clinician, patient or policymaker, all end users of evidence-based healthcare need to execute efficiently and confidently the five key steps of evidence retrieval and application (Figure 1.3). In the chapters which follow, we will look at each of these in more detail and point the reader towards further resources and tools before considering the teaching and learning of evidence-based healthcare.

So what is evidence-based healthcare?

In this book, we will use the term 'evidence-based healthcare'. Is this the same as 'evidence-based medicine'? What about evidence-based practice? Is 'evidence-based' the same as 'evidence-informed'? What is the evidence?

A search on PubMed for articles published in the *Journal of Clinical Epidemiology* reveals 'evidence-based medicine' to be the most popular term closely followed by evidence-based practice (Table 1.5) (16). David Sackett et al. used these two terms interchangeably without ascribing a particular meaning to either term (8). Evidence-based medicine has been attributed to decisions about individuals, while some authors use evidence-based healthcare to describe populations. Another justification for using 'evidence-based healthcare' is that healthcare is not delivered only by doctors. The term 'healthcare' rather than 'medicine' is more inclusive of professionals in nursing and allied health professionals who contribute to research and implementation in healthcare. Many authors acknowledge that all these terms may be used interchangeably (17). A more recent term is 'evidence-informed' (-medicine, -practice and -healthcare). This is intended to acknowledge challenges around implementing evidence and whether it is more realistic to consider evidence informing practice rather than

Table 1.5 Use of 'evidence-based' terms in the titles of articles published in the *Journal of Clinical Epidemiology* (search performed on October 31 2021).

Term	PubMed	*Journal of Clinical Epidemiology*
Evidence-based medicine	4489	16
Evidence-based practice	3693	5
Evidence-based clinical practice	541	1
Evidence-based healthcare (or healthcare)	230	1
'Evidence-based clinical practice' without the word guideline(s)	73	0

Source: Puljak (16)/with permission of Elsevier.

being entirely based on the best available evidence. This has relevance in medical education and how these concepts are framed for healthcare students (18).

The ethical dimension

The aftermath of the Second World War saw several advances to protect the rights of individuals and populations. This extended to medical experimentation and research and will be discussed in Chapter 9. These included the Nuremberg Code, the Declaration of Helsinki, the Belmont Report and the publication in 1996 of Good Clinical Practice, now accepted as the universal standard for the ethical conduct of clinical trials (Table 1.6) (19). No study design should expect to receive approval or findings without ethical consideration. Yet, there remain issues of representation in research which continue to leave historically minoritised and underserved individuals and communities outside the benefits of the best available evidence, and this affects their healthcare. Ethical practice is not a fixed endpoint or destination but one, similar to liberty, self-determination and democracy, where vigilance is imperative. It is not enough to have ethical approval for research but also to ensure that plan is implemented and that the lives of all research participants and the populations whom they represent are all improved by it.

Table 1.6 Thirteen principles of the good clinical practice ethical, scientific and practical standards for research.

- Ethics – clinical trials should be conducted in accordance with the principles of the Declaration of Helsinki
- Trial risk versus trial benefit – risks and inconveniences of a proposed clinical trial should be weighed against the benefits for both participants and wider society. Anticipated benefits should justify the risks
- Trial participants – the rights, safety and well-being of trial participants are the most important considerations and take precedence over the interests of science and wider society
- Information on proposed medicine or intervention – the available information, clinical and nonclinical, about a proposed use of medicine or intervention should be sufficient to justify the proposed trial
- Good-quality trials – should be scientifically robust and explained in a clear, detailed protocol
- Compliance with the study protocol – the study protocol should be reviewed by an independent ethics committee prior to commencement of the study and should then be followed as described
- Medical decisions – all medical care, and all medical decision-making, for study participants should be made by a suitably qualified clinician
- Trial staff – all staff involved in the conduct of a clinical trial should be educated, trained and experienced in their required role. Where necessary, appropriate supervision should be provided
- Informed consent – participants should be given full information to make free and informed consent prior to commencement of the trial
- Clinical trial data – all data related to the trial should be recorded and stored to facilitate accurate reporting, interpretation and verification
- Confidentiality – any information which could identify participants should be protected, including their privacy
- Good manufacturing practice – products used in the investigation and/or intervention should be manufactured, handled and stored in compliance with good practice. They should be stored in accordance with the approved study protocol
- Quality assurance – systems should be implemented in the study design to ensure the quality of all aspects of the trial

Source: Adapted from Biddle K, Blundell A, Sofat N. Understanding clinical research: an introduction. Banbury: Scion Publishing Ltd, 2023 and https://www.ema.europa.eu/en/human-regulatory-overview/research-development/compliance-research-development/good-clinical-practice (accessed August 19 2024).

References

1 Glaszioou, J.A.J. (2017). *A Brief History of Clinical Evidence Updates and Bibliographic Databases.* JLL Bulletin: Commentaries on the History of Treatment Evlauation.

2 (1948). STREPTOMYCIN treatment of pulmonary tuberculosis. *Br Med J* 2 (4582): 769–782.

3 Isaacs, D. and Fitzgerald, D. (1999). Seven alternatives to evidence based medicine. *BMJ* 319 (7225): 1618.

4 Howick, J. (2011). *The Philosophy of Evidence-Based Medicine.* Oxford: Wiley-Blackwell, BMJ Books.

5 Sheridan, D.J. and Julian, D.G. (2016). Achievements and limitations of evidence-based medicine. *J Am Coll Cardiol* 68 (2): 204–213.

6 Thoma, A. and Eaves, F.F. 3rd. (2015). A brief history of evidence-based medicine (EBM) and the contributions of Dr David Sackett. *Aesthet Surg J* 35 (8): Np261–Np263.

7 Canadian Medical Association (1981). How to read clinical journals: I. why to read them and how to start reading them critically. *Can Med Assoc J* 124 (5): 555–558.

8 Sackett, D.L., Rosenberg, W.M., Gray, J.A. et al. (1996). Evidence based medicine: what it is and what it isn't. *BMJ* 312 (7023): 71–72.

9 Sackett, D.L. and Straus, S.E. (1998). Finding and applying evidence during clinical rounds: the "evidence cart". *JAMA* 280 (15): 1336–1338.

10 Straus, S., Eisinga, A., and Sackett, D. (2016). What drove the evidence cart? Bringing the library to the bedside. *J R Soc Med* 109 (6): 241–247.

11 Collaboration C (2017). Cochrane Organisation Dashboard 2017. https://community.cochrane.org/sites/default/files/uploads/inline-files/2017-Dashboard-open_access_16-03-18.pdf (accessed 17 November 2024).

12 Cooper, N., Bartlett, M., Gay, S. et al. (2021). Consensus statement on the content of clinical reasoning curricula in undergraduate medical education. *Med Teach* 43 (2): 152–159.

13 Resnicow, K., Catley, D., Goggin, K. et al. (2022). Shared decision making in health care: theoretical perspectives for why it works and for whom. *Med Decis Mak* 42 (6): 755–764.

14 Oerlemans, A.J.M., Knippenberg, M.L., and Olthuis, G.J. (2021). Learning shared decision-making in clinical practice. *Patient Educ Couns* 104 (5): 1206–1212.

15 Connor, L., Dean, J., McNett, M. et al. (2023). Evidence-based practice improves patient outcomes and healthcare system return on investment: findings from a scoping review. *Worldviews Evid Based Nurs* 20 (1): 6–15.

16 Puljak, L. (2022). The difference between evidence-based medicine, evidence-based (clinical) practice, and evidence-based health care. *J Clin Epidemiol* 142: 311–312.

17 Pattani, R.S.S. (2020). What is EBM?: evidence-based medicine (EBM) toolkit. https://bestpractice.bmj.com/info/toolkit/learn-ebm/what-is-ebm/ (accessed 17 November 2024).

18 Kumah, E.A., McSherry, R., Bettany-Saltikov, J. et al. (2022). Evidence-informed practice versus evidence-based practice educational interventions for improving knowledge, attitudes, understanding, and behavior toward the application of evidence into practice: a comprehensive systematic review of UG student. *Campbell Syst Rev* 18 (2): e1233.

19 Bhatt, A. (2010). Evolution of clinical research: a history before and beyond james lind. *Perspect Clin Res* 1 (1): 6–10.

20 Pallarés-Sanmartín, A., Leiro-Fernández, V., Cebreiro, T.L. et al. (2010). Validity and reliability of the Schamroth sign for the diagnosis of clubbing. *JAMA* 304 (2): 159–161.

21 Vandemergel, X. and Renneboog, B. (2008). Prevalence, aetiologies and significance of clubbing in a department of general internal medicine. *Eur J Intern Med* 19 (5): 325–329.

CHAPTER 2

Identifying Clinical Questions

Raj Himatshih Babla

Division of Medical Sciences and Graduate Entry Medicine, University of Nottingham, Nottingham, UK
Clinical Implementation Lead, Stoneygate Centre for Empathic Healthcare, University of Leicester, Leicester, UK

OVERVIEW

- Clinical questions emerge from patient interactions, clinical texts and educational settings.
- Identifying an answerable question is the first step in evidence-based healthcare.
- Clinical questions may be either background or foreground questions.
- Clinical questions are usually linked to aetiology, diagnosis, therapy, prognosis and prevention.
- Using the PICO framework to structure clinical questions facilitates evidence retrieval.
- Finding appropriate evidence based on the clinical question is key to improving clinical expertise and patient care.

Introduction

Clinical questions arise from various settings, including direct patient encounters, clinical reading or educational environments such as meetings, lectures and workshops. Effectively identifying these questions is crucial and involves understanding patient care contexts, specific patient needs and principles of evidence-based medicine (EBM). The goal is to come back to the individual patient (or population) to derive the best possible outcome for them.

In EBM, identifying an answerable question is the first of five steps (1). A structured approach to formulating clinical questions includes identifying the clinical problem, recognising the type of question being asked and using frameworks like PICO (patient/problem, intervention, comparison and outcome) to guide the research to answer the question (2).

The process involves gathering a comprehensive patient history, performing a physical examination and synthesising information to form a clear clinical picture. Engaging with patients to understand their expectations and needs is also essential.

A clinical question arises for several reasons. For example, uncertainty about the best treatment option for a particular condition, especially when guidelines are unclear or conflicting. Clinicians may also encounter unusual symptoms or rare diseases that require deeper investigation to ensure accurate diagnosis and appropriate management. Additionally, staying up to date with the latest research and evidence can highlight innovative approaches or therapies, improving patient outcomes. Furthermore, patient-specific factors, such as comorbidities or unique social circumstances, can create complex scenarios that require tailored, evidence-based solutions.

Once clinical questions are identified, conducting focused literature searches and critically appraising the evidence help integrate findings with clinical expertise and patient preferences, guiding better patient care (Figure 2.1) (3).

Clinical background questions versus foreground questions

When formulating clinical questions, it is essential to distinguish between background and foreground questions. This differentiation helps in understanding the nature of the information being sought and guides the appropriate approach for finding answers.

What are background questions?

These are typically broader, foundational questions, aimed at enhancing general knowledge about a condition or treatment. They often consider basic or general information and are commonly asked by those new to a topic or needing a refresh on the information (4).

These questions typically have two key components (5):
1 A question root (who, what, where, when, why, how) + a verb (5)
2 An aspect of the disorder, test, treatment or other healthcare aspects (5)

These questions are usually answered by consulting medical textbooks, reviewing articles, clinical guidelines or reputable online resources (Box 2.1).

ABC of Evidence-Based Healthcare, First Edition. Edited by John Frain.
© 2025 John Frain. Published 2025 by John Wiley & Sons Ltd.

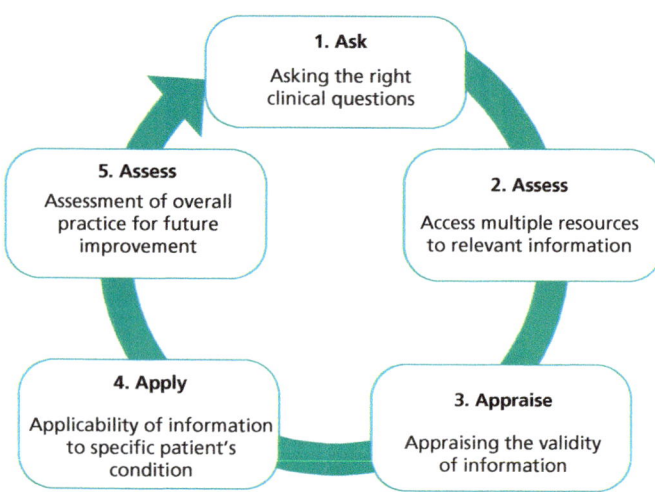

Figure 2.1 The five-step guide to practise evidence-based medicine. *Source:* Muhamad et al. (3)/JMIR Publications/CC BY 4.0.

Box 2.1 **Examples of background questions**

- Who is predisposed to diabetes mellitus?
- What causes heart failure?
- Where is the hippocampus found?
- When do complications of kidney disease usually occur?
- Why do people develop back pain?
- How does smoking affect the body?

What are foreground questions?

These are usually more detailed and specific. They focus on precise clinical decisions or actions. Often, these are asked by clinicians seeking an evidence-based answer to support decisions in patient care (4).

These questions are best structured using the PICO framework to ensure they are focused and answerable (2). Foreground questions are answered through systematic searches of current, peer-reviewed medical literature (see Chapter 3) (Box 2.2).

Understanding the difference between background and foreground clinical questions is crucial for effective evidence-based practice. Background questions provide the necessary foundation of knowledge, while foreground questions drive the specific, evidence-based decisions required for optimal patient care (4). Utilising the appropriate resources and frameworks for each type of question ensures clinicians can more effectively find and apply the best available evidence in their practice in a timely manner.

Where do clinical questions come from?

Clinical questions may arise from direct patient contact whilst reading clinical texts or in a learning environment, such as a clinical lecture or workshop (1). Effectively identifying clinical questions involves several aspects, including understanding the context of patient care, the specific needs of the patient and the principles of EBM (1).

Box 2.2 **Key differences in background and foreground questions**

- Scope:
  - Background questions – broad and general, aimed at understanding basic concepts and general knowledge (4).
  - Foreground questions – specific and detailed, aimed at informing clinical decisions and actions (4).
- Complexity:
  - Background questions – usually simpler, providing a foundation or context.
  - Foreground questions – more complex (11), often requiring detailed and precise answers based on latest research.
- Use in clinical practice:
  - Background questions – used for gaining a general understanding (4), often by medical students or clinicians encountering a new topic.
  - Foreground questions – used for making specific clinical decisions (11), often by practising clinicians seeking evidence to support patient care.
- Answers:
  - Background questions – answered by textbooks, review articles and general medical resources.
  - Foreground questions – answered by primary research articles, systematic reviews, clinical guidelines and other evidence-based resources.

The following is a structured approach to formulating clinical questions:

Identifying the clinical problem

The clinical problem could relate to the patient's symptoms, diagnosis, treatment options or prognostic concern. This may well be linked to the patient's main concern or issue, though not necessarily. It may be an area we are unfamiliar with, therefore posing a further question for us. A common way this has been described is as Patient Unmet Needs (PUNS) and Doctor's Educational Needs (DENS) (Figure 2.2) (6).

At times, there can be a disconnect between the patients' expectations and a clinician's agenda, so it can help to clarify the question at hand. An example of the potential differing perspectives is seen in Box 2.3.

Identifying a clinical problem involves several key components. At each step, a clinical question could be revealed, and not all steps may be necessary for each patient with regard to a specific question becoming clear.

Gather a comprehensive history

To identify a clinical problem, we must start by collecting detailed, clinically relevant information about the patient. This includes the history of the current presentation, medication history, family history, social history and so forth.

Perform a thorough physical exam

An examination can provide vital clues about the patient's presentation. It may be normal, which can also add intrigue, where you may have thought an abnormality may have been expected.

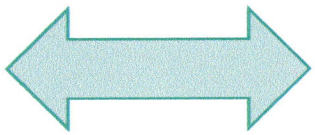

Patient unmet needs	Doctor's educational need
Due to lack of knowledge or skill on the doctor's part, consultations may have a patient's unmet need.	Identified from consultations where knowledge or skill may be improved.

Figure 2.2 PUNs and DENs.

Box 2.3 **Patient versus doctor perspectives – an example of peripheral arterial disease**

Patient's perspective
- Symptom relief – often the primary concern for patients who may be experiencing pain, cramping and discomfort during walking or exercise.
- Quality of life – patients are likely to prioritise the ability to perform everyday activities without limitations.
- Treatment side effects – concern about potential side effects of either medicines or surgery.
- Non-invasive option – preference for non-invasive to avoid surgery and associated risks.
- Psychological impact – concerns about the emotional and psychological effects of living with a chronic condition and how it affects their mental health.

Doctor's perspective
- Disease severity – assessing severity through history, examination and diagnostic tests to determine the best course of action.
- Treatment efficacy – evaluating the effectiveness of various treatment options, including lifestyle modifications, medications and surgery.
- Risk factors – identifying and managing risk factors such as smoking, diabetes, hypertension and high cholesterol to prevent disease progression and complications.
- Monitoring and follow-up – establishing a plan for regular monitoring and follow-up.
- Multidisciplinary approach – coordinating care with other healthcare professionals, including vascular surgeons, cardiologists and physical therapists, to provide holistic patient care.

Use of Investigations

These may not be necessary for all patients. Examples include laboratory tests – blood tests, urine analysis and swabs; imaging – X-rays, CT scans and ultrasounds; specialised tests – ECGs, endoscopies and biopsies.

Patient engagement

Appropriately engaging with the patient is a key step in considering the aim of the clinical question at hand (see Chapter 8). Are there different expectations from the patient compared to your thoughts on the situation? Do they agree with the question to consider the treatment required? It may be that more than one clinical question may be helpful to answer, from the clinician and from the patient.

Types of clinical questions (6, 7)

Ask yourself the type of clinical question you are considering, as this will influence the type of evidence you search for. This may be apparent as you go through the initial steps mentioned earlier or become clearer after you have had time to contemplate (Box 2.4).

Using the PICO framework (2, 8)

After clarifying the type of question we are asking, it is helpful to structure this to help us efficiently answer the question.

There are several question frameworks which can be used (Box 2.5). However, the PICO framework (2) has been widely used and researched and has proven efficacy (9). It aids us in structuring clinical questions to make them easier to research and answer. We can use this, formally or informally, to guide our understanding:

- *Patient/Problem* – Describe the patient or problem in detail. Include specific characteristics, including age, gender, ethnicity and specific health conditions or disease (2).
- *Intervention* – Specify the main area of focus you are considering, for example, aetiology, diagnostic tests and treatment options (2).
- *Comparison* – Identify any potential comparisons to the intervention, which may be considered. These include placebos, no treatment or a different treatment (2).
- *Outcome* – Define desired or expected outcomes. This could be an improvement in symptoms, a better outcome from treatment or overall health improvement (2).

This framework was developed in the early 1990s as part of the EBM movement (2). We use this framework to give a structured method to formulate a clinical question and conduct literature searches, making EBM simpler, more accessible and systematic (Box 2.6).

Box 2.4 **Types of clinical questions**

- Aetiology/harm – Questions about the causes of disease or effects of harmful agents.
- Diagnosis – Questions about accuracy of diagnosis, including from history taking or diagnostic tests.
- Therapy – Questions about options and effectiveness of treatments.
- Prognosis – Questions about the potential course or outcome of a disease.
- Prevention – Questions about strategies to prevent disease.

Source: Adapted from Icahn School of Medicine at Mount Sinai (7).

Box 2.5 **PICO, PICOT and PIO frameworks**

There are a range of frameworks to aid in answering clinical questions. These are three commonly used tools.

The PICO framework is a widely used tool for formulating clinical questions and structuring research queries in evidence-based practice. It focuses on the four main components outlined earlier.

The PICOT framework (4), like the PICO framework, adds a component to specify the timeframe for the intervention and outcomes. This helps to narrow down the search for evidence and focuses on the duration over which the outcomes are measured.

The PIO framework is a simplified version of PICO. It is often used for broader questions, such as public health research, when a comparison may not be necessary.

Source: Adapted from Stillwell et al. (4).

Box 2.6 **Why use the PICO framework?**

1 Clarity and focus (8) – PICO helps formulate clear, focused clinical questions that are specific and answerable. This focus is crucial for conducting efficient and effective literature searches.
2 Efficiency (9) in research – By breaking down a clinical question into its basic components, PICO makes it easier to identify relevant studies and evidence, saving time and resources in the research process.
3 Improving search strategy (2) – PICO facilitates in providing keywords for database searches, improving the precision and relevance of the search results.
4 Enhances critical appraisal (12) – It helps provide a clear framework for evaluating and comparing studies, ensuring conclusions are based on high-quality evidence.
5 Supports evidence-based practice (2) – PICO aligns well with the principles of EBM, aiming to integrate clinical expertise with the best available evidence.

Finding evidence

Once a specific clinical question has been formulated, we need to consider where we are and how and where to research the answer. This is usually done by entering search terms into a medical database such as PubMed or the Cochrane Library. If the question being asked is well structured, the search terms are easier to derive using the keywords in your PICO framework (Box 2.7). There are several credible databases, such as PubMed and Cochrane Library. This is discussed further in Chapter 3.

Appraise, apply and evaluate the evidence

Once you have found relevant studies, critically appraise their validity, relevance and applicability to your patient's situation (Chapter 7). Integrate the evidence with your clinical expertise and patient preferences. Evaluate the outcomes after applying the evidence-based intervention and adjust as necessary (Chapter 8).

Box 2.7 **Examples of using PICO to derive search terms**

a In patients with *chronic migraines* (P), does *acupuncture* (I), compared to *no treatment* (C), reduce the *frequency* of *migraine* attacks (O)?
  i. Keywords – chronic migraines, migraine sufferers; acupuncture, needle therapy; no treatment, placebo; reduce migraine frequency, decreased migraines.
b In patients with *suspected deep vein thrombosis* (DVT) (P), is a *D-dimer* test (I), compared to *Doppler* ultrasound (C), more effective in confirming the *diagnosis of DVT* (O)?
  i. Keywords – suspected DVT, DVT, deep vein thrombosis, blood clot; D-dimer; Doppler ultrasound; confirm DVT, diagnose DVT, diagnose deep vein thrombosis.
c In *adolescents* using *social media* (P), does *excessive screen time* (I), compared to *limited screen time* (C), increase the risk of developing *anxiety disorders* (O)?
  i. Keywords – adolescents, teenagers, youth, social media use; screen time screen exposure; limited screen time, low screen usage; anxiety, anxiety disorders, mental health.

Examples of differing types of clinical questions using the aforementioned structured approach

As noted earlier, there are different types of clinical questions which may form after the question is identified. Following are worked examples of these different types of clinical questions using the PICO framework.

Aetiology/harm

Patient background – a 61-year-old female patient has been advised it is best to reduce or quit smoking prior to her elective knee replacement surgery. She has previously failed in the past to quit smoking; however, she is keen to try again. She has not tried nicotine replacement products previously. She has a strong family history of cardiovascular disease; however, she has no history of this herself. Due to her family history, she is worried nicotine replacement products may increase her risk of cardiovascular disease rather than quitting without their use.

Using the PICO framework, we can formulate an answerable question:

Do smokers (P) who have used long-term nicotine replacement therapy (NRT) to quit smoking (I) compared to those without using any NRT (C) have a lower incidence of cardiovascular events (O)?

Diagnosis

Patient background – a 12-year-old child attends the Accident and Emergency Department with their parents. They have been complaining of central abdominal pain which has moved to the right iliac fossa. Appendicitis is suspected. You are unsure how accurate an ultrasound would be compared to a computed tomography (CT) scan to diagnose this patient.

Clinical question – For children presenting with symptoms of appendicitis (P), is an ultrasound (I), in comparison to a CT scan (C), an accurate diagnostic tool (O)?

Therapy

Patient background – An 82-year-old male patient with a background of hypertension and hypercholesterolaemia attends for an annual hypertension review. He is taking two therapies as per the National Institute for Health and Care Excellence (NICE) guidance for his hypertension and a statin. He has not made many lifestyle changes in the past despite advice. His home blood pressure readings are still raised above the expected threshold, and he is not keen to add further medication. A discussion around lifestyle changes resurfaces, and he is keen to understand more about whether a low-sodium diet will really make that much impact given his age.

Clinical question – For patients with hypertension over 80 years of age (P), will implementing a low-sodium diet (I), compared to making no changes to salt intake (C), cause a reduction in blood pressure levels (O)?

Prognosis

Patient background – A 29-year-old female patient who has been diagnosed with early-stage breast cancer is due to undergo genetic testing to determine the risk to any future children. She has no other past medical history and was adopted, so she is unaware of any family history. She does not smoke and only drinks alcohol on special occasions. She wants to know whether the presence of any specific genetic markers will influence 10-year survival rates compared to patients without the marker.

Clinical question – In patients with localised early-stage breast cancer (P), does having specific genetic markers (I), compared to no genetic markers (C), affect the 10-year survival rate after diagnosis (O)?

Prevention

Patient background – A 48-year-old male is aware that bowel screening in the United Kingdom is available to those who are 50–74 years old. However, he would like to reduce the risk of bowel cancer for himself if possible. This is following a friend who was diagnosed with end-stage bowel cancer, and they did not have any screening done, as they were too young for the screening programme. The patient has not had any symptoms suggestive of bowel cancer, however, recalls reading in a newspaper that aspirin can reduce the risk of bowel cancer, along with cardiovascular events, so is keen to consider this.

Clinical question – In adults with an average risk of colorectal cancer (P), does taking low-dose aspirin for a minimum of five years (I), compared to no aspirin use (C), reduce the incidence of colorectal cancer (O)?

Health economics in clinical questions

A further important aspect is the consideration of health economics in clinical questions, as it affects our clinical practice, decision-making and influences the allocation of resources. When formulating clinical questions, considering the economic implications can provide a more comprehensive understanding of the value and feasibility of different interventions.

Integrating health economics into the PICO framework (10)

Making some adaptations to the PICO framework, as detailed earlier, we can integrate health economics to provide a more holistic view:

- *Patient/Problem* – Consider the economic burden of the disease or condition on the patient and healthcare system.
- *Intervention* – Include the costs associated with the intervention, such as treatment expenses, implementation costs and long-term financial impact.
- *Comparison* – Evaluate the costs of alternative interventions or the lack of intervention.
- *Outcome* – Incorporate economic outcomes such as cost savings, cost-effectiveness ratios and improvements in QALYs (quality-adjusted life years).

Incorporating health economics into clinical questions (10)

There are a range of areas where considering health economics in clinical questions can be beneficial (Box 2.8).

Integrating health economics into clinical questions ensures a comprehensive evaluation of interventions, considering not only their clinical effectiveness but also their economic impact. This approach helps in making informed decisions that optimise resource use, improve patient outcomes and ensure sustainable healthcare practices. By incorporating cost-effectiveness, budget impact, cost-benefit analysis and QALYs into the PICO framework, clinicians can

---

Box 2.8 Examples of PICO integrating health economics into clinical questions

1 Cost-effectiveness analysis (10, 13) – this compares the relative costs and outcomes of different types of action.
   a. Example – In adults with chronic back pain (P), is physical therapy (I), compared to surgical intervention (C), more cost-effective in improving functional outcomes (O)?
2 Budget impact analysis (14) – this estimates the financial consequences of adopting a new intervention within a specific budget.
   a. Example – In a primary care setting (P), does the introduction of a new telemedicine programme (I), compared to traditional in-person visits (C), have a lower impact on the annual healthcare budget (O)?
3 Cost-benefit analysis (13) – this compares the benefits of an intervention in monetary terms to its costings.
   a. Example – In a hospital (P), does implementing a new infection control protocol (I), compared to standard practices (C), result in net financial savings (O) due to reduced infection rates?
4 Quality-adjusted life years (13) – this measures the value of health outcomes by combining the quantity and quality of life.
   a. Example – In patients with end-stage renal disease (P), does kidney transplantation (I), compared to continued dialysis (C), provide more QALYs over 10 years?

address both clinical and economic aspects of patient care, contributing to more effective and efficient healthcare delivery.

The impact of answering clinical questions

It may help to consider how the concepts discussed earlier can be applied and expanded in your professional journey.

Applying evidence-based practice in daily clinical practice

- Begin implementing structured question formulation using the PICO framework regularly when encountering clinical dilemmas. Engaging with colleagues in case discussions and journal clubs to practise formulating and answering clinical questions together.
- Routine literature searches – develop a habit of conducting regular literature searches using databases like PubMed and Cochrane Library and others mentioned. Use evidence summaries from trusted resources such as UpToDate or ClinicalKey to quickly integrate findings into clinical practice.

Engaging in continuous learning and professional development

- Professional growth – consider pursuing additional training or certification in EBM, clinical research or health economics to deepen your expertise. This can include participating in workshops, webinars and conferences focusing on the latest advancements in your field.
- Mentorship and collaboration – consider working with experienced clinicians proficient in evidence-based practice. Learning from their experiences can provide valuable insights for efficient and effective practice.

Integrating health economics into clinical decision-making

1 Economic evaluations in clinical practice – begin to consider the economic aspects of clinical decisions by incorporating them into your practice. Use tools and resources that provide economic evaluations of interventions, helping you balance clinical effectiveness with economic viability.
2 Advocate for cost-effective interventions in your clinical setting by presenting data and evidence to support economically sound practices. Consider engaging in discussions about healthcare resource allocation and the impact of economic considerations on patient care outcomes.

Future research and quality improvement

1 Conducting and participating in research – get involved in clinical research projects that aim to answer important clinical questions and contribute to the evidence case. Collaborate with research teams and academic institutions.
2 Quality improvement initiatives – within clinical settings, lead or participate in quality improvement initiatives within your healthcare setting. Use the principles of evidence-based practice to identify areas for improvement and implement change.

Monitor and evaluate the outcomes of these initiatives to ensure they lead to meaningful improvement in patient care and resource utilisation.

Summary

Formulating and addressing clinical questions using evidence-based practice is an essential tool in modern-day medical practice. It is a skill that combines understanding patient needs with a structured approach to finding and applying evidence. The process is critical to high-quality patient care, requiring a robust evidence base to inform decisions. This chapter highlights the importance of identifying clinical questions, utilising structured approaches like the PICO framework and, additionally, considering health economics. By consistently applying these methods, clinicians can improve their understanding and interpretation of patient care, leading to better outcomes. Ongoing education and participation in research or quality improvement exercises are areas which can further contribute to EBM, which will enhance patient care and effective healthcare resource application.

References

1 Swanson, J.A., Schmitz, D., and Chung, K.C. (2010). How to practice evidence-based medicine. *Plast Reconstr Surg* 126 (1): 286–294. https://doi.org/10.1097/PRS.0b013e3181dc54ee. PMID: 20224459; PMCID: PMC4389891.

2 Richardson, W.S., Wilson, M.C., Nishikawa, J., and Hayward, R.S. (1995). The well-built clinical question: a key to evidence-based decisions. *ACP (American College of Physicians) J Club* 123 (3): A12–A13. PMID: 7582737.

3 Muhamad, N.A., Selvarajah, V., Dharmaratne, A. et al. (2022). Online searching as a practice for evidence-based medicine in the neonatal intensive care unit, university of Malaya medical center, Malaysia: cross-sectional study. *JMIR Form Res* 6 (4): e30687. https://doi.org/10.2196/30687. PMID: 35384844; PMCID: PMC9021944.

4 Stillwell, S.B., Fineout-Overholt, E., Melnyk, B.M., and Williamson, K.M. (2010). Evidence-based practice, step by step: asking the clinical question: a key step in evidence-based practice. *AJN, American Journal of Nursing* 110 (3): 58–61. https://doi.org/10.1097/01.NAJ.0000368959.11129.79.

5 Winona State University (2024). Evidence based practice toolkit. https://libguides.winona.edu/ebptoolkit/EBP (accessed 12 August 2024).

6 Eve, E. (2020). PUNs and DENs: a model for reflective learning. *InnovAiT* 13 (3): 189–190. https://doi.org/10.1177/1755738019883313.

7 Icahn School of Medicine at Mount Sinai (2009). Evidence based medicine: the PICO framework. https://libguides.mssm.edu/ebm/ebp_pico (accessed 12 July 2024).

8 Schardt, C., Adams, M.B., Owens, T. et al. (2007). Utilization of the PICO framework to improve searching PubMed for clinical questions. *BMC Med Inform Decis Mak* 7: 16. https://doi.org/10.1186/1472-6947-7-16.

9 Huang, X., Lin, J., and Demner-Fushman, D. (2006). Evaluation of PICO as a knowledge representation for clinical questions. *AMIA Annu Symp Proc* 2006: 359–363. PMID: 17238363; PMCID: PMC1839740.

10 Mathes, T., Walgenbach, M., Antoine, S.-L. et al. (2014). Methods for systematic reviews of health economic evaluations: a systematic review, comparison, and synthesis of method literature. *Med Decis Mak* 34 (7): 826–840. https://doi.org/10.1177/0272989X14526470.

11 University of Canberra (2020). Evidence-based practice in health. https://canberra.libguides.com/c.php?g=599346&p=4149723 (accessed 12 August 2024).

12 Straus, S.E., Richardson, W.S., Glasziou, P., and Haynes, R.B. (2018). *Evidence-based Medicine: How to Practice and Teach EBM*, 5e. Philadelphia, PA: Elsevier Churchill Livingstone.

13 Oslo University Hospital. Health economics. https://www.ous-research.no/home/healtheconomics/FAQ/23748 (accessed 12 August 2024).

14 Sullivan, S.D., Mauskopf, J.A., Augustovski, F. et al. (2014). Budget impact analysis-principles of good practice: report of the ISPOR 2012 budget impact analysis good practice II task force. *Value Health* 17 (1): 5–14. https://doi.org/10.1016/j.jval.2013.08.2291. Epub 2013 Dec 13. PMID: 24438712.

CHAPTER 3

Finding the Evidence

Alistair Hewins¹ and John Frain²

¹ Final Year Graduate Entry Medical Student, University of Nottingham, Nottingham, UK
² Division of Medical Sciences and Graduate Entry Medicine, University of Nottingham, Nottingham, UK

OVERVIEW

- Medical information, including journal articles, can be found easily searching the internet.
- Understanding how evidence is stored and classified in controlled databases enables retrieval of higher-quality evidence in greater volumes.
- The researcher may need to retrieve all available evidence on a topic.
- The busy clinician needs to find high-quality, pre-appraised evidence which summarises a topic quickly and efficiently.
- Both types of retrieval require skills to ensure relevant, appropriate evidence is selected.
- Demonstrating how evidence was retrieved is included in reporting standards for study designs, including systematic literature reviews.

Where is the evidence?

Articles published in medical journals are accessible in controlled databases on the internet. Some are freely accessible (e.g. PubMed), whilst others require access from within an academic institution or healthcare provider (Table 3.1). The database enables retrieval of article titles and abstracts. Access beyond this depends on the database used and whether the article is 'open access' (Box 3.1). Library services in an institution usually have subscriptions to journals commonly required by individuals working or studying in the organisation. This allows articles to be downloaded, usually in a PDF format. Library services often provide training in searching skills. Where a research project requires a comprehensive literature search, it is sensible to involve a librarian in the team or discuss requirements with them before undertaking a search. Resources for learning and practising search skills can be found in the Useful Tools section.

What is a database?

A database is an organised collection of data for storing, managing and retrieving information about a person, group or topic. A database is controlled by a database management system (DBMS).

Modern databases have management systems enabling storage and user interaction from a range of devices (handheld, iPad, desktop, home, work and mobile devices). This enables retrieval of information through searches.

Each record (e.g. a scientific or medical paper) is tagged with several identifiers facilitating its easy retrieval during searches, for example, the topic, title, author, journal, year of publication or page numbers. The user interface includes a search facility to identify papers of interest to answer a particular topic. Articles are retrieved using keywords, with the most recently published at the top of the list, though other priorities can be selected.

Medical summaries and databases

The prolific growth in clinical evidence and published literature needs to be accessible to clinicians. The development of indexing, association and computers has enabled the development of bibliographic databases (1). They form a key part of medical literature and include alert bulletins or evidence updates, which may also be retrieved from online databases (1).

Articles published in journals are indexed in databases which include those journals. PubMed and Embase are updated daily, others twice weekly and others less frequently. Any article published in a peer-reviewed journal included within a database is indexed so it can be retrieved through an online search. Often, letters responding to an article, comments and corrections may also be found linked to the original article.

What is peer review?

Peer review is a method of quality assurance of publications in healthcare journals. On submission for publication, every article is reviewed by the editorial board to ensure it meets the requirements and scope of the journal in question. If suitable, it is sent for review by the author's professional peers. They assess the quality of the literature review, design and execution of the study, quality of data collection, statistical analysis and interpretation of results.

Table 3.1 Commonly used bibliographic databases.

Database	Content	Link	Comments
AMED	Allied and complementary medicine including palliative care	https://www.ebsco.com/products/research-databases/allied-and-complementary-medicine-database-amed	500 journals index; abstracts dating back to 1995
BNI	Nursing, midwifery and community care	https://proquest.libguides.com/BNI/content	Indexes most popular English language journals; mainly the United Kingdom with small selection from the United States and Australia
CINAHL	Nursing and allied health	https://www.ebsco.com/products/research-databases/cinahl-database	Content includes 3360 active index and abstracted journals including 3320 active peer-reviewed indexed and abstracted journals
Cochrane Library	Database of systematic reviews (CDSR)	https://www.cochranelibrary.com	Contains high-quality systematic reviews. Cochrane MeSH browser is useful for identifying MeSH terms for use in a search strategy
Embase	Biomedical and pharmaceutical health	https://www.elsevier.com/en-gb/products/embase	Facilitates systematic reviews using a PICO format. Provides evidence on drug adverse events and medical device regulations
Emcare	Nursing, midwifery and allied health	https://www.wolterskluwer.com/en/solutions/ovid/ovid-emcare-14007	Produced by Elsevier and covering 1995 onwards. Indexes 3700 current international journals and contains over 5 million records
HMIC	Healthcare management	https://ospguides.ovid.com/OSPguides/hmicdb.htm	Official publications, journal articles and grey literature relating to health and social care management
Medline	Biomedical, life sciences, allied health and preclinical sciences literature	https://www.nlm.nih.gov/medline/medline_overview.html	National Library of Medicine (NLM) contains over 31 million journal articles. Records are indexed with MeSH headings
Psychinfo	Psychology, behavioural sciences and related disciplines	https://www.apa.org/pubs/databases/psycinfo	Over 5.5 million records from 2400 journals. AI and machine-learning-powered assistance
PubMed	Free database including Medline, life science and biomedical sources	https://pubmed.ncbi.nlm.nih.gov	Public open access database since 1997. Contains over 37 million articles
Social Policy and Practice	Behavioural and social sciences, social work and public health	http://www.spandp.net	Contains information from six UK collections on social policy and practice resources

Box 3.1 **What is an 'open-access' article?**

Open-access articles and books have been published and made freely available online. They are publicly available and do not require a subscription. They can be used free of charge. The published material can be reused without permission from the author or publisher, provided the correct citation to the original article is included. Open access provides greater opportunity for an article to be read and for subsequent researchers and authors to build upon the work. Articles are more likely to be cited by others and by a wider range of authors.

Since an author (or institution) pays an article processing charge (APC), this adds to the costs of funding a project. Journals publishing articles open-access rely on APCs as a funding stream. This leaves them open to criticism of undermining the peer review process and publication bias. These have been addressed, and around one-third of the articles are now published as open access.

An assessment is made of the new article's contribution to the existing literature, and a recommendation is made on whether it should be published. Reviewers are usually experts in the article's topic. Any article retrieved from a controlled medical database will have gone through this process prior to publication.

Can't I just use Google it?

It is common to 'just Google it'. For information of little consequence (e.g. Which football club is the most successful? What other films has this actor been in?), the truth of the answer has little if any consequence. For information affecting a patient's diagnosis and/or treatment, incorrect information may have dire consequences.

'Googling it' is common among both patients and healthcare professionals. Google searches may provide patients with useful and reliable information about the origin and problems associated with a disease (2). However, general searches with Google are likely to be unreliable when describing treatments. Among many reasons for training in evidence-based healthcare is clinicians' need to direct the patient towards reliable and up-to-date sources of information (e.g. reliable patient information leaflets) (Chapter 8). Many patients browse the internet for information prior to seeing a clinician and after receiving a diagnosis. Multiple studies report a lack of accuracy and reliability of the internet for obtaining health information (3, 4). Information about treatment is often incomplete, written by non-experts and may have commercial objectives (2). There is no correlation between search results on Google appearing high on a list and the quality of their information (5). Search results are not ranked on the basis of quality, and in some cases, the first results seen may be sponsored content given a higher priority to be seen first by the user.

Google is a commercial search engine and not designed to be an authoritative and unbiased source of health information. Results may not be the most up-to-date, evidence-based or high-quality information. Misinformation and disinformation sources are difficult to spot. Sites may be unsuitable for lay users and have poor readability. The sheer number of search results (e.g. supplements in cancer) may be daunting and make discrimination difficult (5).

Sites are often linked to commercial websites or product placements. There are often related advertisements attached. Search results may be related to the geographical location of the user and based on priorities, including commercial.

What about Google Scholar?

Google Scholar (GS) enables broad searching of academic or scholarly literature. This includes articles, theses, books and abstracts. Publishers include academic sources, professional societies and universities. While guidance within the evidence-based medicine (EBM) world is that GS should not be used in isolation from recognised databases, it can retrieve a broad range of results. A review of 29 systematic reviews published in the Cochrane Database of Systematic Reviews or *Journal of the American Medical Association* in 2009 found all studies included in these reviews would have been found by GS had no other database been used (6). A prospective comparison of databases found GS to have slightly less coverage than Embase and Medline combined (97.2% versus 97.5%) (7). Search results on GS have been limited to the first 1000, and advanced searches are more difficult. GS does not support data downloads, and clearer indexing guidelines are required. Any comprehensive literature search, such as for a systematic literature review (SLR), will involve several databases. Within this, GS has a qualified place.

Hierarchies of evidence – the evidence pyramids

Before considering how to search and retrieve evidence, it is worth considering how evidence may be categorised. Not all evidence is created equal in quality or relevance. This results from aspects such as study design and how the research is reported for publication. Assessing the quality of research forms part of critical appraisal (Chapter 7). However, it is time-efficient to understand where best and what type of evidence to seek. Understanding hierarchies of evidence can aid clinical decision-making. There are two evidence pyramids to consider:

The pyramid of studies

This hierarchy applies more to scientific research than to clinical diagnosis, decision-making or management (Figure 3.1). A top-down approach to the pyramid should be taken with an initial search made for a well-conducted SLR. If one is not available, the researcher moves down to the next level of evidence and so on. Several versions of this hierarchy are published. Whilst they vary slightly, the principle is the same – studies are ranked on the strength and precision of their methodologies. Use of a pyramid to visualise this conveys the reality that evidence at the lower levels is more voluminous than the higher ones.

Unfiltered information represents original research studies, such as case reports and randomised controlled trials (RCTs), which have not been synthesised or incorporated into SLRs or guidelines. Filtered information includes SLRs and meta-analyses. Data from studies included in SLRs are reviewed prior to inclusion based on strict criteria. By reviewing and aggregating large numbers of studies, SLRs can portray a wider picture of the current research. Since the retrieval and evaluation have been done already, these are helpful to busy clinicians. Filtered resources are more likely to provide a definitive answer to a clinical question.

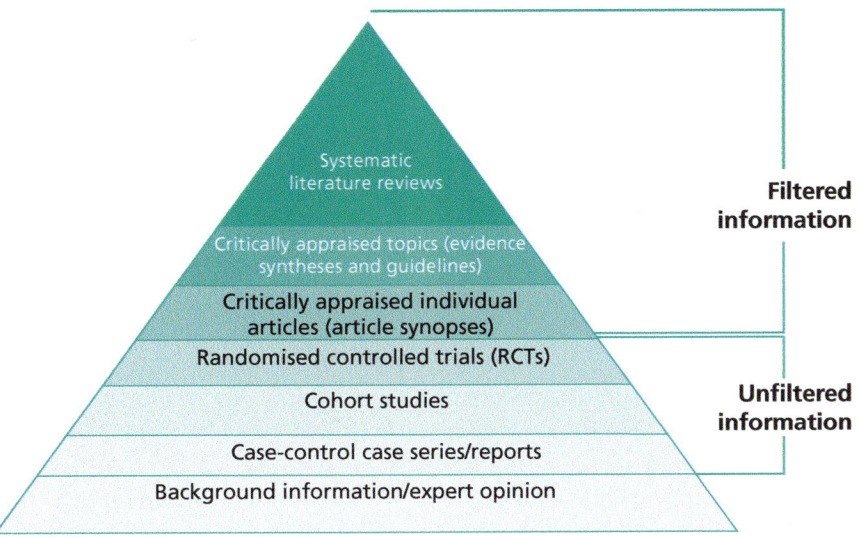

Figure 3.1 Hierarchy of evidence for scientific research. *Source:* Adapted from https://openmd.com/guide/levels-of-evidence.

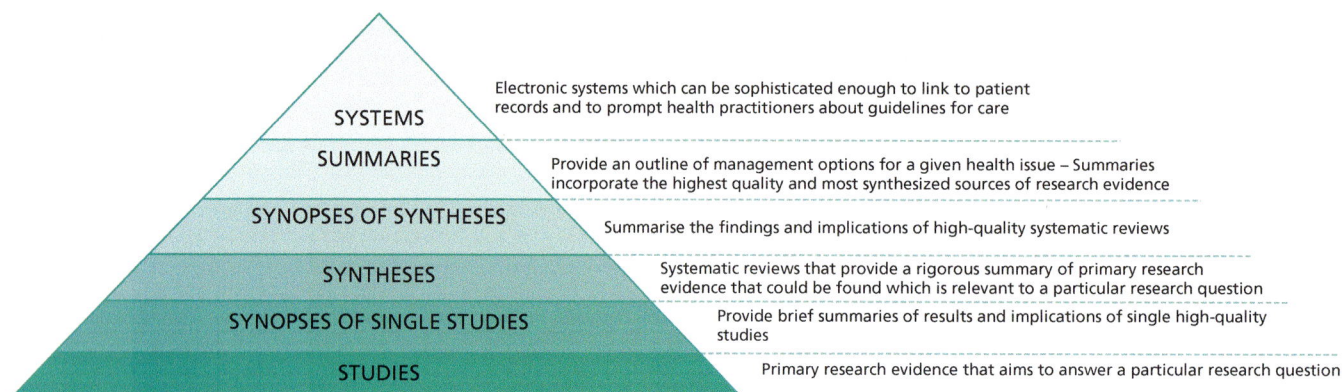

Figure 3.2 The 6-S pyramid of research evidence. *Source*: Adapted from: ebn.bmj.com/content/12/4/99.2.

The '6-S Pyramid' (8)

This is a classification aimed at the end user of EBM resources (e.g. busy clinicians) needing information about diagnosis and management quickly. The resources contain evidence to help clinicians answer foreground questions about individual patients, situations or research topics (Figure 3.2) (see Chapter 2). Again, the intention is to use a top-down approach for retrieving evidence at the highest possible level of the pyramid (Table 3.2) (9).

Search strategies

The clinical question should drive the strategy behind an information search. Use of a standardised format for asking questions was discussed in Chapter 2. Benefits of a standardised format (e.g. PICO, PICOT) enable the clinician to specifically define components of the clinical problem. Clinical questions define what kind of information will best answer the question. Well-formulated questions may also assist in identifying outcomes to be evaluated once the evidence is applied to individual patients or groups.

Getting started

Searching should start with broad search terms to establish the volume of information which may be available on the chosen topic. More focused search terms should then be used, specific to each component of the PICO or similarly structured research question. Finally, by combining broad and focused search terms, retrieval of articles relevant to the research question can be maximised. Initially, it may take a novice several attempts to see what works and what is less effective.

Deriving search terms

Search terms can be either individual words such as 'asthma' or 'diabetes' or combinations of words such as 'left ventricular systolic dysfunction' or 'congestive cardiac failure'.

Use of a PICO (or PICOT or PCO format) facilitates a more structured search for relevant information. The elements of the PICO should contain ideally all the key terms for which you are searching and will indicate where each of the information needs lie in relation to the greater whole (Box 3.2). Keywords, similar words or synonyms should all be used as search terms in the

Table 3.2 Resources for evidence-based practice.

Systems	Decision-support systems which integrate with individual patient records (e.g. Ardens for SystemOne and EMIS Web in the UK National Health Service)
Summaries	**Clinical practice guidelines**
	NICE Clinical Guidelines – National Institute for Health and Care Excellence, UK
	British Thoracic Society – Asthma Guidelines
	Evidence-based texts
	Dynamed
	BMJ Best Practice
	Clinical Overviews (Clinical Key)
	Evidence-Based Physical Diagnosis, fifth Edition 2021
Synopses of syntheses	NHS Centre for Reviews and Dissemination (CRD)
	Cochrane Evidence Summaries
	Cochrane Podcasts
	OrthoEvidence
	HealthEvidence.org
	Evidence-based abstract journals
	Evidence-Based Medicine
	ACP Journal Club
	Evidence-Based Obstetrics and Gynaecology
	Evidence-Based Mental Health
	Cancer Treatment Reviews
	Evidence-Based Healthcare and Public Health
	Evidence-Based Nursing
	JAMA – Rational Clinical Examination
Syntheses	Cochrane Library
	Cochrane Neonatal Reviews
	EPC Evidence Reports
	The Cochrane Collaboration
Synopses of single studies	Evidence-Based Medicine
	ACP Journal Club
	OrthoEvidence
	Evidence-Based Obstetrics and Gynaecology
	Evidence-Based Mental Health
	Cancer Treatment Reviews
	Evidence-Based Healthcare and Public Health
	Evidence-Based Nursing
Single studies	**Article databases**
	CINAHL
	Ovid Databases – Medline, EMBASE, PsychINFO, AMED
	PubMed
	ProQuest Nursing and Allied Health Source
	Health Services (HSR) Queries
	Clinical queries
	PubMed Clinical Queries
	CINAHL Clinical Queries
	OVID Clinical Queries

Box 3.2 **Deriving Search Terms from a PICO Question**

		Search terms
Problem (patient)	Adult patient presenting with knee pain without a pre-existing diagnosis of an ACL injury	'anterior cruciate ligament' 'ACL'
Intervention	Anterior drawer test	'anterior drawer test' 'anterior drawer exam'
Control	Lachman test	'Lachman test' 'Lachman exam'
Outcome	Presence/absence of knee injury (confirmed by MRI)	'ACL injury' 'ACL tear'

database. Use of only acronyms and abbreviations should be avoided, at least initially, as they may not be the terms used in abstracts and may thus be missed. Both long and short terms should be used instead (e.g. 'anterior cruciate ligament' and 'ACL').

Deriving effective search terms can be challenging and is the most difficult part of the literature search. Following a systematic approach such as a PICO format enables the researcher to create search terms specific to the clinical question and hopefully minimises time spent reviewing unrelated or inappropriate information.

Exploding your search

With your initial search, you should not start too narrowly; otherwise, you may miss relevant evidence (Figure 3.3). It is better to identify as many papers as possible and then narrow these down to produce a focused search. This is called 'exploding your search' and means you will identify the keyword and all the associated narrower terms simultaneously. Consequently, all articles indexed using narrow terms and listed below the broader term are included in the search. Although this may identify too many results, it reduces the risk of missing something important.

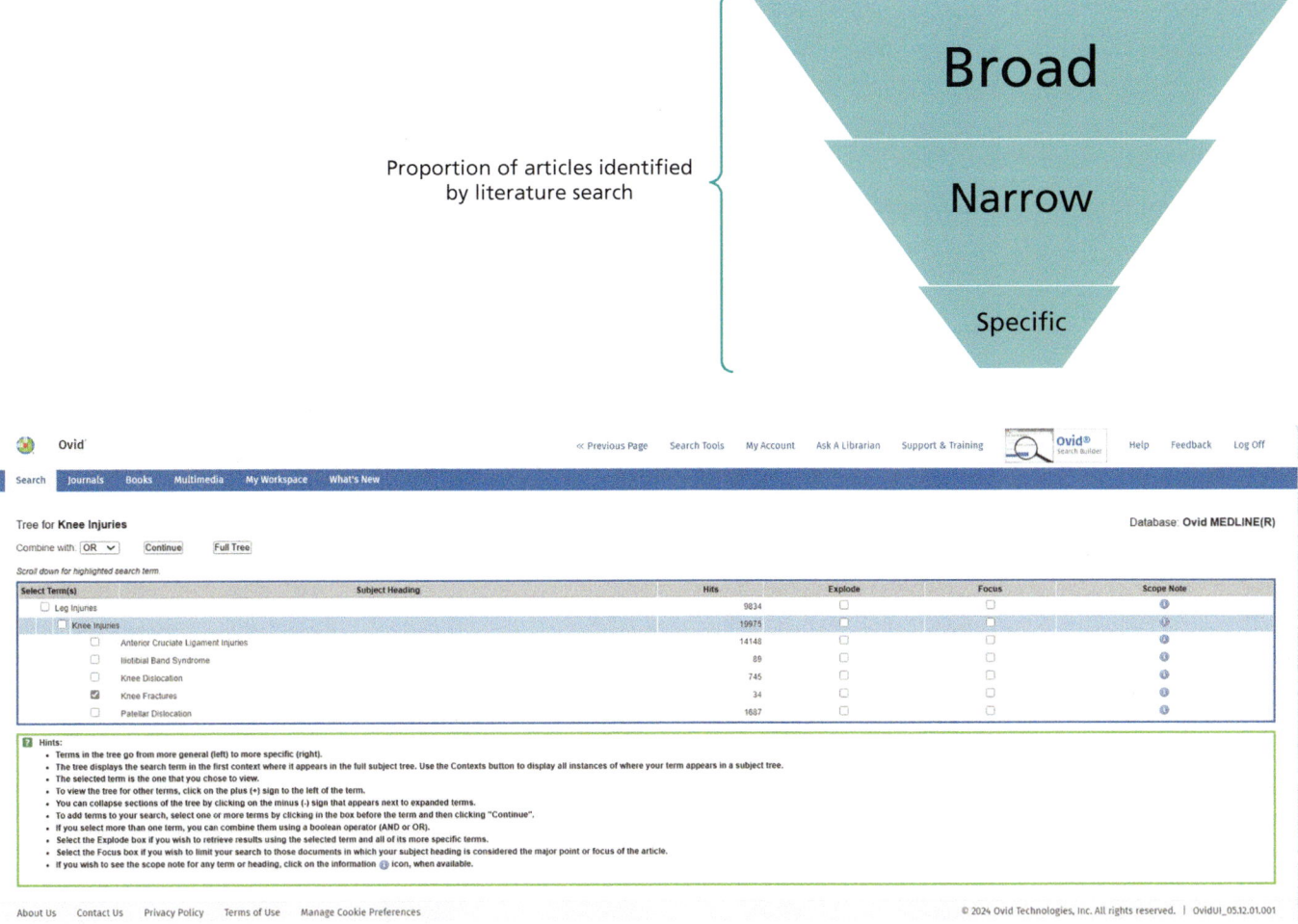

Proportion of articles identified by literature search

Broad

Narrow

Specific

Figure 3.3 Process of broad-narrow search terms/articles identified. By 'exploding' the Medical Subject Heading (MeSH) 'knee injuries' in the Ovid® search engine's tree function, we can see the multiple topics that are indexed underneath. Articles will be indexed to the database with one or more of these topics and can therefore be utilised to broaden or narrow a literature search. For example, by selecting the 'knee fractures' topic, one should be able to identify articles specific to that condition whilst avoiding picking up articles specific to unrelated ones such as 'Iliotibial Band Syndrome'. Familiarising oneself with the tree function in Ovid® or the Cochrane Library MeSH browser is a good method to derive effective search terms.

Focusing the search

Filters can be used to refine a search and get more specific results. Publication date is useful for identifying up-to-date publications (e.g. last 5 or 10 years). Subheadings can also be used alongside index terms to narrow the search. Indexers assign keywords to articles to facilitate their retrieval from databases. These words can also be weighted by labelling them as major headings and represent the main concepts of an article. This further facilitates focusing of a search. Examples include the 'Title and/or Abstract' filter, which matches search terms to text in the title or abstract. In contrast, the 'Text Word' filter identifies search terms in the entirety of the document, including references. This filter often returns a large number of hits and should be used with a specific objective (e.g. identifying niche outcome measures that may not be reported in the abstract).

Limiting a search to titles only

The title may not mention a keyword crucial to the search. Where searches are limited to titles only, an important article may be missed. For example, searching 'Treat depression' using the 'Title' filter returns ~200 results, whereas using the same search term in the 'Title and/or Abstract' filter returns over 1600 results. A full text search may pick the name of a disease mentioned in the text even though the article is not about the disease itself but an entirely different topic.

Using Boolean operators

Boolean operators are tools used in combination with search terms. Boolean operators allow a search engine within a database to limit, narrow or broaden search results to identify content which is most relevant to the research question. The advanced search builder in PubMed enables intuitive searching using Boolean operators (Figure 3.4). The commonest operators are AND, OR and NOT. Note the operators must all be typed in capitals to be used to focus a search strategy (OVID is an exception) (Table 3.3). Research results at each stage are tabulated in a user-friendly manner and facilitate a combination of search strands.

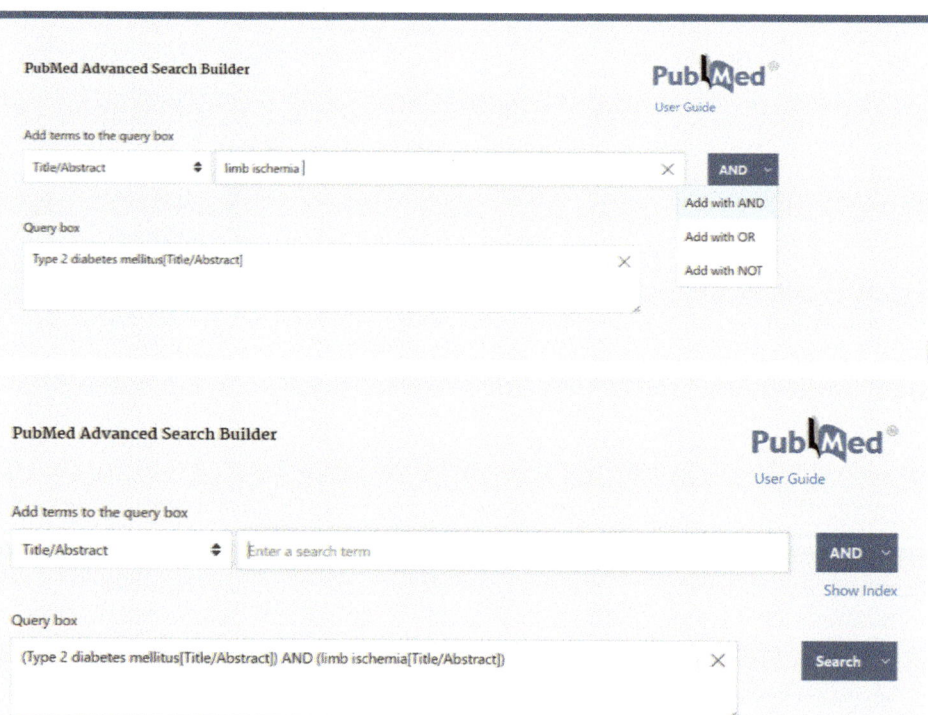

Figure 3.4 Building a search with Boolean operators.

Table 3.3 Examples of search results using Boolean operators.

	Search terms	Hits
1	'chronic obstructive pulmonary disease' (Title/Abstract)	65 538
2	'COPD' (Title/Abstract)	62 666
3	'chronic obstructive pulmonary disease' OR 'COPD' (Title/Abstract)	85.023
4	'chronic obstructive pulmonary disease' AND 'COPD' (Title/Abstract)	43 181
5	((smoker [Title/Abstract]) OR (smoking [Title/Abstract]) OR (smokes [Title/ Abstract])	286 152
6	#3 NOT #5	73 057

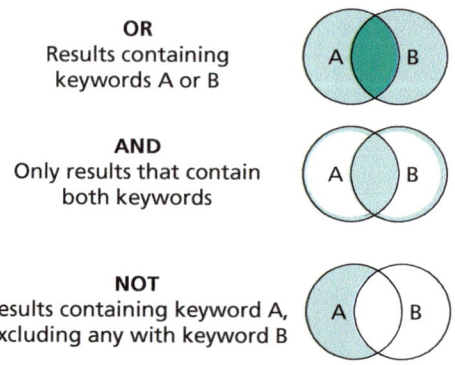

OR
Results containing keywords A or B

AND
Only results that contain both keywords

NOT
Results containing keyword A, excluding any with keyword B

Table 3.4 Tools for focusing literature searches.

Tool	Definition	Example
Quotation marks ' '	Provides results with the exact phrase rather than a search based on the individual words in the phrase. Search engines are not usually case-sensitive, e.g. diabetes and Diabetes.	'type 2 diabetes mellitus'
Parentheses ( )	Searches often include multiple keywords and/or multiple Boolean operators. Use of parentheses enables the search engine to group them in a way most relevant for the research question.	(type 2 diabetes mellitus OR T2DM)
Truncation	It is the use of * after use of a main stem. The search will then return all possible endings of that word; for example, cardio * returns cardiology, cardiovascular and cardiothoracic. A variety of truncation symbols are used, including ?, * and +.	
Wild card	A wild card symbol within a word will return the possible characters that can be substituted. For example, wom(#)n will return woman and women. Common wild card symbols include the hash and ?.	
Stemming	Most search terms will 'stem' search words/terms. Stemming removes suffixes such as -s, -ing and -ed. These variations are retrieved automatically when stem words are searched.	
Synonyms	Search engines might expand searches by using thesaurus to match search words to other words with the same meaning.	
Plus (+)	Use a plus (+) symbol before a term that must appear in the search results.	
Stopwords	Common words such as 'and', 'this' and 'also' are not indexed. These stop words are words that, if indexed, could occur in every article in a database if the word is used in a search.	
Limit words	This can be achieved by, for example, limiting to human subjects, publication type, date, language of publication, etc.	

AND

AND allows a search to be narrowed to find all results having BOTH/ALL search terms present – contains all the keywords present.

OR

The OR operator retrieves all results with EITHER/ANY of the search terms used – provides results containing either keyword.

NOT

NOT tells the search engine to exclude results containing a particular search term – provides results containing the first keyword but not the second. NOT needs to be used carefully as there may be papers which use both terms and to exclude one term may in fact exclude a paper one wishes to find (e.g. Asthma NOT emphysema).

Other search tools are displayed in Table 3.4.

Thesaurus

These are used in databases (e.g. Medline) to facilitate effective searching. A shared vocabulary is used to index information from different journals. This is done by grouping related concepts under

Box 3.3 **Search terms – worked example using the original PICO**

PICO	#	Search terms	Hits
	1	Anterior cruciate ligament injury (MeSH Terms)	14122
Problem	2	'ACL tear' (Title/Abstract) OR 'anterior cruciate ligament tear' (Title/Abstract) OR 'ACL rupture' (Title/Abstract) OR 'anterior cruciate ligament rupture' (Title/Abstract)	3121
Combine	3	#1 OR #2	15229
Intervention/comparator	4	'Lachman test' (Title/Abstract) OR 'anterior drawer test' (Title/Abstract)	1189
	5	'Diagnosis'(Title/Abstract) OR 'detect' OR 'identify' (Title/Abstract) OR 'rule-in'(Title/Abstract) OR 'rule-out'(Title/Abstract)	3751831
Outcome	6	'specificity'(Title/Abstract) OR 'sensitivity'(Title/Abstract) OR 'validity'(Title/Abstract) OR 'diagnostic accuracy' (Title/Abstract)	1564250
Combine	7	#4 OR #5 OR #6	4944571
	8	#3 AND #7	3267
	9	('2021/08/01' (Date – Publication): '2024/07/18' (Date – Publication) AND #8	802

a single preferred term. As a result, all indexers use the same standard terms to describe a subject area, regardless of the term authors have chosen to use. It contains keywords, definitions of those keywords and cross-references between keywords. The National Library of Medicine (NLM) uses a thesaurus called Medical Subject Headings (MeSH). MeSH is a hierarchically organised vocabulary produced by the NLM. It is used for indexing, cataloguing and searching of biomedical and health-related information. MeSH includes the subject headings appearing in Medline/PubMed, the NLM catalogue and other NLM databases. The Cochrane MeSH browser is a reliable source of MeSH terms, which can facilitate identification of useful search terms. MeSH contains over 27000 items. Each keyword represents a single concept found in the medical literature. For most MeSH terms, there will be broader, narrower and related terms to consider for selection.

These tips can be used then to facilitate a detailed search using the original PICO question (Box 3.3).

Comprehensive search strategies

These use different databases to ensure all relevant information is retrieved, which is particularly important in research such as SLRs and meta-analyses. It is essential that the same approach is taken across each database. Protocols for SLRs should include how the literature search will be undertaken. The published article should report the search strategy according to a standard protocol (e.g. PRISMA) (Figure 3.5) (11).

All searches should include the following steps (12):

1 Determine a clear and focused question.
2 Describe the articles that can answer the question.

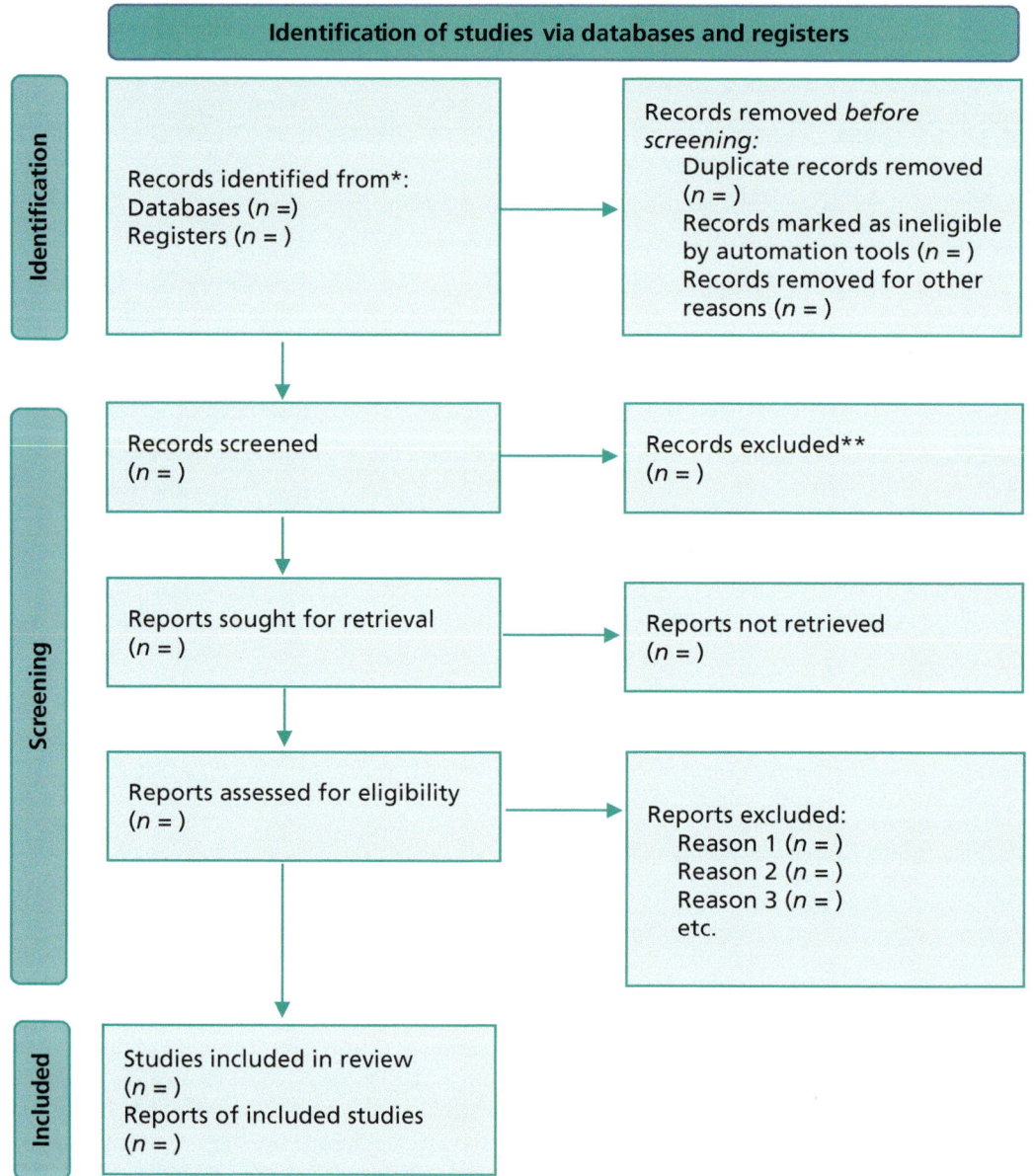

Figure 3.5 PRISMA 2020 flow diagram for new systematic reviews which included searches of databases and registers only. *Source:* Page et al. (10)/BMJ Publishing Group Ltd/CC BY 4.0. *Consider, if feasible to do so, reporting the number of records identified from each database or register searched (rather than the total number across all databases/registers). **If automation tools were used, indicate how many records were excluded by a human and how many were excluded by automation tools.

3 Decide which key concepts address the different elements of the question.
4 Decide which elements should be used for the best results.
5 Choose an appropriate database and interface to start with.
6 Document the search process in a text document.
7 Identify appropriate index terms in the thesaurus of the first database.
8 Identify synonyms in the thesaurus.
9 Add variations in search terms.
10 Use database-appropriate syntax with parentheses, Boolean operators and field codes.
11 Optimise the search.
12 Evaluate the initial results.
13 Check for errors.
14 Translate to other databases.
15 Test and reiterate.

Different research methods may have different levels of quality, validity and reliability. This creates the evidence pyramid. Evidence near the top of the pyramid (Figures 3.1 and 3.2) is likely to have undergone critical appraisal and therefore will be more applicable to answering a research question whilst being less prone to bias. Guidelines are commonly accepted by clinicians as being well-researched and informative for clinical practice. However, they cannot be applied in every scenario. Alternative evidence sources to inform clinical decision-making are described next.

Systematic review

If suitable guidelines are not available, an SLR on the topic of interest should be sought. These are published across many journal types. The clinical queries facility in PubMed has a way of retrieving these. The best database of these is the Cochrane Database of Systematic Reviews. These SLRs are accepted as the highest standard in evidence-based healthcare. The Cochrane library specialises in reviews assessing the effectiveness of interventions for prevention, treatment and rehabilitation and the accuracy of diagnostic tests.

Primary research papers

If we are unable to find a systematic review, we will need to look for one or more original research papers. These are indexed in databases such as Medline, PubMed and Embase. Medline is a large database of clinical papers with over 30 million references to 5200 biomedical journals published in over 40 languages (https://www.nlm.nih.gov/medline/medline_overview.html). This can also be searched using PubMed, which is open to use by all. Checking references lists in recent guidelines, reviews and primary sources is helpful, as authors will have recently searched the literature when writing these.

Internet searches

If nothing can be found from searching medical databases, searches of internet engines such as Google, Yahoo or Bing can be tried. As previously discussed, internet searches of non-medical/scientific databases may not return good-quality, reliable evidence and therefore should be used with caution. Here, quotation marks can be used to search exact phrases (such as 'off-label treatment of [insert condition]'). This will help narrow the search and avoid returning too many results. Key sources of information to be considered in this instance are patient advocacy groups (https://www.genomics education.hee.nhs.uk/genotes/knowledge-hub/rare-disease-patient-advocacy-groups/#the-benefits-of-pags-for-medical-professionals), which may offer insights into alternative management strategies or research opportunities. Also, press releases from pharmaceutical companies may contain snippets of information relating to clinical trials which are either still ongoing or not ready to publish their findings yet.

Grey literature

This is any material which does not find its way into the standard medical databases. It includes government reports, policy documents, patents, academic theses and conference abstracts. Many organisations make grey literature available. There are search engines which specialise in it (Box 3.4). Grey literature may not have been peer reviewed, and this may make it less reliable. However, a comprehensive literature search for an evidence synthesis (e.g. systematic review) should include relevant grey literature.

Selecting studies

Once evidence has been identified, a list of titles and abstracts will have been produced. These need to be screened for: (i) Is the topic relevant to the research question being asked? (ii) What is the study design used, and is it suitable to the question being asked? (iii) Is it of sufficient quality for our purposes? All these topics will be included in subsequent chapters.

Box 3.4 Sources of grey literature

- Mednar
- WorldWideScience.org
- PsychEXTRA
- OAIster
- Google
- ProQuest
- Clinical Trial Registries
- OpenGrey (SIGLE)
- Congresses and conferences for various specialities
- Patient advocacy groups

Limitations of the evidence pyramid

The evidence pyramid places emphasis on the study design rather than how well the design was implemented (Chapter 7) and how it aligns to other studies of the same issue. A well-conducted cohort study may be better than a poor RCT. Where conditions are rare, the sample sizes required for an RCT may not be possible, and case-control studies are more appropriate.

Randomisation (see Chapter 4) may not always be possible, or it may be unethical, e.g. high cholesterol versus normal cholesterol diet or drinking alcohol versus not drinking alcohol. Additionally, use of a placebo in control groups may hinder recruitment efforts in cancer trials where patient survival is dependent on treatment.

The evidence hierarchy does not apply in qualitative research, where methodology has a different approach to quantitative research. The pyramid should not be used rigidly; it may not be suitable for questions requiring different research methods but should serve as a guide to identifying reliable sources of information to further one's understanding of the literature.

Tips on abstract screening

Three-step approach

1 Read the abstract to see if it is relevant to our question and if the approach is suitable.
2 Does the background accord with what we know? Are the method and sampling strategy appropriate for the clinical question? Studies in controlled settings with defined samples need to be relevant to our own patients. Review the results and draw your own conclusions. Use validated tools to critically appraise and decide if the results are reliable. If the results are reliable and we agree with the conclusions, this may be enough to commit us to a change in our own practice.
3 Where the findings may be significant for a change in our own practice, a full critical appraisal is necessary (Chapter 7). Letters to the editor may be helpful in picking up flaws in the research.

Reporting a search

The literature search should be explained in the methods section of a systematic review and done in accordance with an appropriate guideline such as PRISMA (11). All steps undertaken should

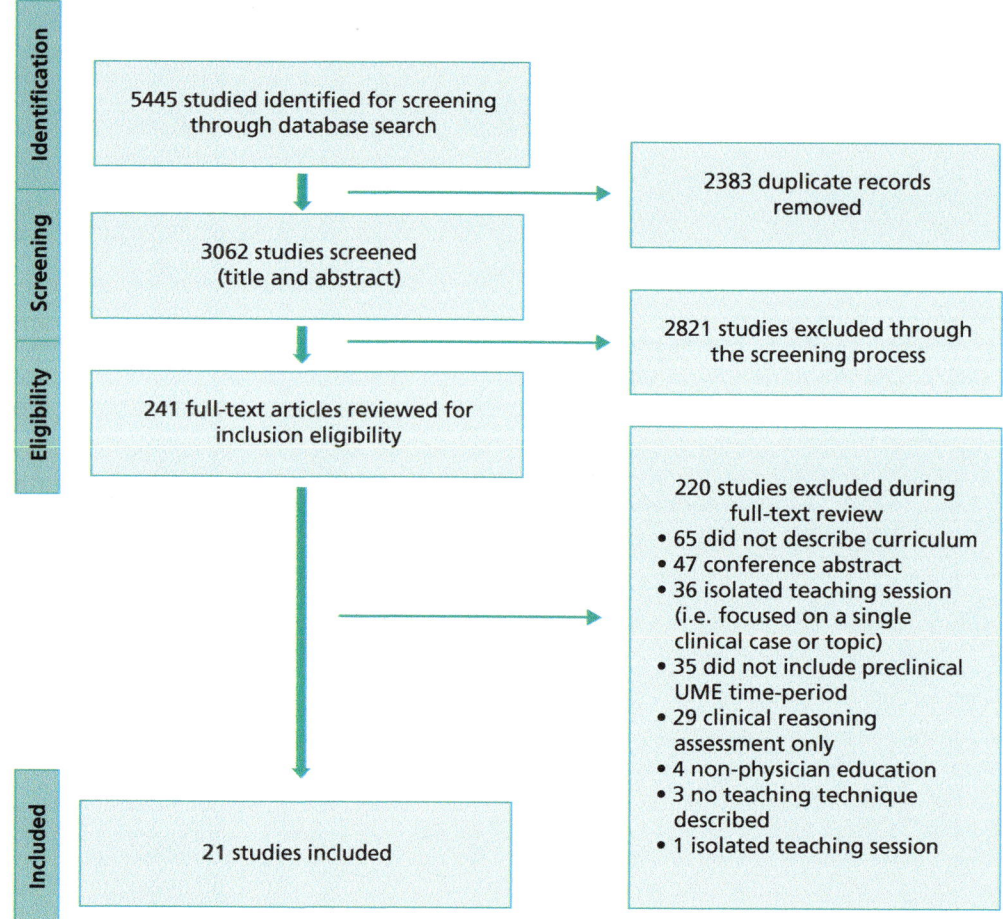

Figure 3.6 PRISMA flowchart for a scoping review on clinical reasoning education in preclinical undergraduate medical education. *Source:* Hawks et al. (13)/with permission of Wolters Kluwer Health, Inc.

be listed in a clear, precise manner. The timeframe of the search should be stated (e.g. articles published in the last five years), the databases and/or sources of evidence that were used in the search (e.g. Medline and relevant conference proceedings); examples of search terms used should be reported and all relevant inclusion and exclusion criteria that were used to screen and ultimately select the evidence used. A flow diagram (Figure 3.6) should be drawn up to illustrate the steps of the search and can also be used to highlight themes of the identified evidence.

References

1 Glasziou, J.A.J. (2017). *A Brief History of Cloinical Evidence Updates and Bibliographic Databases.* JLL Bulletin: Commentaries on the History of Treatment Evlauation.

2 Kothari, M. and Moolani, S. (2015). Reliability of "Google" for obtaining medical information. *Indian J Ophthalmol* 63 (3): 267–269.

3 Morr, S., Shanti, N., Carrer, A. et al. (2010). Quality of information concerning cervical disc herniation on the Internet. *Spine J* 10 (4): 350–354.

4 Yeung, T.M. and Mortensen, N.J. (2012). Assessment of the quality of patient-orientated Internet information on surgery for diverticular disease. *Dis Colon Rectum* 55 (1): 85–89.

5 Cai, H.C., King, L.E., and Dwyer, J.T. (2021). Using the Google™ search engine for health information: is there a problem? case study: supplements for cancer. *Curr Dev Nutr* 5 (2): nzab002.

6 Gehanno, J.F., Rollin, L., and Darmoni, S. (2013). Is the coverage of Google Scholar enough to be used alone for systematic reviews. *BMC Med Inform Decis Mak* 13: 7.

7 Bramer, W.M., Giustini, D., and Kramer, B.M. (2016). Comparing the coverage, recall, and precision of searches for 120 systematic reviews in Embase, MEDLINE, and Google Scholar: a prospective study. *Syst Rev* 5: 39.

8 DiCenso, A., Bayley, L., and Haynes, R.B. (2009). Editorial: accessing pre-appraised evidence: fine-tuning the 5S model into a 6S model. *ACP J Club* 151 (6): 2–3.

9 University M (2024). *Resources for Evidence-Based Practice: The 6S.* Pyramid Hamilton, Ontario: McMaster University. https://hslmcmaster.libguides.com/ebm.

10 Page, M.J., McKenzie, J.E., Bossuyt, P.M. et al. (2021). The PRISMA 2020 statement: an updated guideline for reporting systematic reviews. *BMJ* 372: n71.

11 PRISMA (2020). Prisma.org. https://www.prisma-statement.org.

12 Bramer, W.M., de Jonge, G.B., Rethlefsen, M.L. et al. (2018). A systematic approach to searching: an efficient and complete method to develop literature searches. *J Med Libr Assoc* 106 (4): 531–541.

13 Hawks, M.K., Maciuba, J.M., Merkebu, J. et al. (2023). Clinical reasoning curricula in preclinical undergraduate medical education: a scoping review. *Acad Med* 98 (8): 958–965.

CHAPTER 4

Principles of Study Design

John Frain

Division of Medical Sciences and Graduate Entry Medicine, University of Nottingham, Nottingham, UK

OVERVIEW

- Research is a planned and systematic activity which discovers new facts or identifies relationships between facts.
- A research study design is a systematic plan for carrying out research effectively and efficiently.
- A research study design may be descriptive, analytical or experimental.
- Study design is important as it ensures the correct methodology is used to answer the research question.
- Good study design increases the credibility, validity and applicability of the study results.
- Understanding the choice of a study design is essential to assess the quality of evidence.

Introduction

'Research is a planned and systematic activity which attempts to discover new facts or to identify relationships between facts. It attempts to achieve this in an objective manner which will ensure the data obtained can be generalised, that is, can be applied to a wider range of situations than the one studied and that the data are not influenced by the conscious or unconscious bias of the investigator or any other extraneous factors' (1).

Research study design

The two initial questions to consider are (Figure 4.1) (2):
- Is the study descriptive (non-analytic) or analytic?
- Which design or method is being used?

Non-analytic studies

A non-analytic or descriptive study describes what is happening in a population (e.g. the prevalence, incidence of a disease or experience of a group). It does not try to quantify or explain the variables described or their relationship to one another. Descriptive studies include case reports, case series, qualitative studies and survey (cross-sectional) studies, which measure the frequency of several

factors and hence the size of the problem (Box 4.1). A descriptive study may identify an area for further research (3). It may also include analytic work (e.g. comparing factors). Observational studies investigate and record exposures (such as interventions or risk factors) and observe outcomes (such as disease) as they occur.

Analytic studies (4)

An analytic study attempts to measure the relationship between two factors. This is commonly the effect of an intervention (I) or an exposure (E) on an outcome (O). To quantify the effect, we will need to know the rate of outcomes in both a comparison (C) group and the intervention (I) or exposed (E) group. Whether the study changes a factor in the E group or uses an intervention in an I group determines whether the study is observational (researcher's involvement is passive) or experimental (researcher's involvement is active) (Box 4.2) (5). In analytic observational studies, the researcher simply measures the exposure or treatments of the groups. Analytical observational studies include case-control studies, cohort studies and some population (cross-sectional). These studies all include matched groups of subjects and assess associations between exposures and outcomes.

Experimental studies (6)

In experimental studies, the researcher manipulates the exposure by allocating subjects either to an intervention/exposure group or to a control group who do not receive the intervention or exposure. Subjects are allocated to one of two or more groups to receive an intervention or exposure and then followed up under carefully controlled conditions. Such controlled trials, particularly if randomised and blinded, have the potential to control for most of the biases that can occur in scientific studies. Whether this occurs depends on the quality of the study design and implementation (Box 4.3) (7).

What type of study am I reading?

Appraising study design is covered in Chapter 7. However, the overall design of a study should be immediately identifiable from three questions (Box 4.4). The type of clinical question being asked also provides a clue to the study design most appropriate for an answer (Table 4.1).

ABC of Evidence-Based Healthcare, First Edition. Edited by John Frain.
© 2025 John Frain. Published 2025 by John Wiley & Sons Ltd.

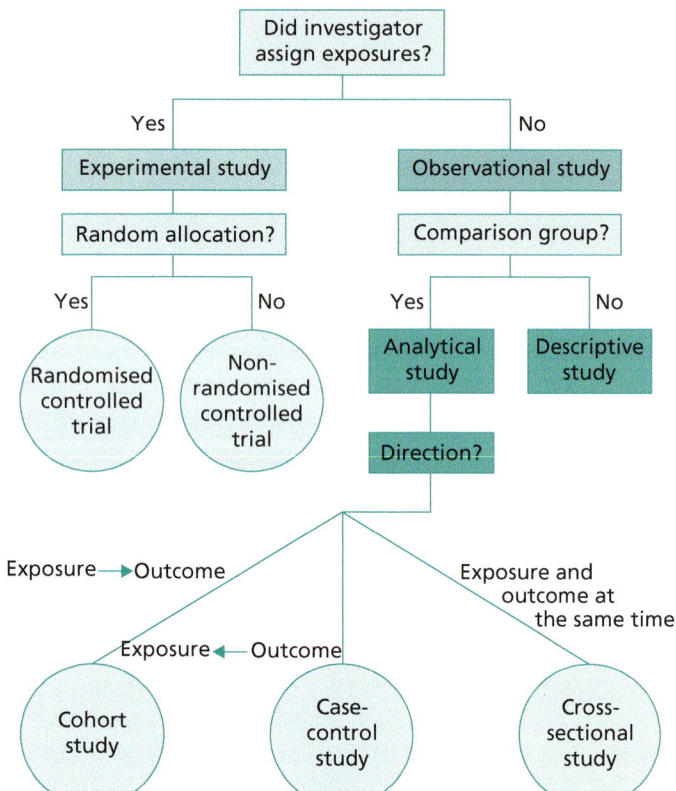

Figure 4.1 Flow chart to assess the study design which has been used. *Source:* Grimes and Schulz (2)/with permission of Elsevier.

Box 4.1 **Descriptive study of association between quality of care and empathy and burnout in primary care (3)**

A cross-sectional study of family physicians and nurses was conducted in Spain. Empathy and burnout were measured using the Jefferson Empathy Scale and the Maslach Burnout Inventory. Quality of care was measured using Quality Standard Indicator (QSI) scores. Practitioners with low empathy had higher QSI scores than those with high empathy (672.8 versus 654.4), while those with high burnout had higher scores than those with low burnout (702 versus 671). Burnout and empathy did not significantly influence quality of care delivery in primary care centres. More studies are needed to investigate the unexpected finding that physicians and nurses with higher levels of burnout provide higher quality care.

Source: Yuguero et al. (3)/Springer Nature/CC BY 4.0.

We should finally note that studies can incorporate several design elements. For example, the control arm of a randomised trial may also be used as a cohort study, and the baseline measures of a cohort study may be used as a cross-sectional study.

Accounting for bias in study design

To ensure studies are valid and trustworthy, it is essential to account for bias from the outset. Bias is any tendency which prevents unprejudiced consideration of a research question (8).

Box 4.2 **Maternal vitamin D status affects bone growth in early childhood – a prospective cohort study**

Eighty-seven children were followed up from birth to 14 months with data on maternal vitamin D status during pregnancy. Background data were collected by questionnaire and a three-day food record. The children were divided into two groups (Low D and High D) based on maternal vitamin D status during pregnancy. Both groups were given vitamin D supplements during the study. There was greater gain in bone mineral content in the Low D group than the High D group of children ($p = 0.032$). Postnatal vitamin D supplements improved vitamin status but only partly eliminated differences in bone variables induced by maternal vitamin D status during pregnancy. Further attention should be paid to improving maternal vitamin D status during pregnancy.

Source: Adapted from Viljakainen et al. (5).

Box 4.3 **A randomised trial of intensive versus standard blood pressure control (7)**

The most appropriate targets for systolic blood pressure to reduce morbidity and mortality among people without diabetes were uncertain. This study randomly assigned 9361 people with a systolic blood pressure of 130 mmHg or higher and an increased cardiovascular risk to a systolic blood pressure target of either under 120 mmHg (intensive treatment) or less than 140 mmHg (standard treatment). The primary outcome was myocardial infarction, other cardiovascular conditions or death from cardiovascular causes. All-cause mortality was significantly lower in the intensive treatment group (hazard ratio, 0.73; 95% CI, 0.60–0.90; $P = 0.003$). Rates of serious adverse events were higher in the intensive-treatment group compared with the standard-treatment group.

Source: Adapted from Wright et al. (7).

Box 4.4 **What is the design of this study I am reading?**

Q1 What did this study aim to achieve?
 1 Describe a population (PO) – descriptive.
 2 Quantify the relationship between factors (e.g. PICO questions) – analytic.
Q2 If an analytic study, was the intervention randomly allocated?
 1 Yes? Randomised controlled trial (RCT)
 2 No? Observational study
Q3 When were the study outcomes determined?
 1 Before the study was commenced (RCT)
 2 Sometime after the exposure or intervention (cohort study)
 3 At the same time as the exposure or intervention (cross-sectional study or survey)
 4 Before the exposure was determined (case-control study) ('retrospective study' based on recall of the exposure)

Table 4.1 Suitable study designs for clinical questions.

Clinical question	Explanation of research question	Appropriate study designs
Prevention	What is the effectiveness of an intervention or exposure in preventing morbidity or mortality from a condition? Are there any potential harms?	Randomised controlled trials Prospective study
Aetiology/harm (causation)	What is the effect of this intervention or exposure on a patient?	Cohort Case-control Case series
Diagnosis	What is the ability of a test or procedure to differentiate between those who have or do not have a condition?	RCT Cohort study
Therapy (treatment)	Is this intervention effective in improving outcomes in sick patients or patients suffering from a condition? (Interventions can include medications, surgery, procedures, lifestyle changes and talking therapies)	RCTs
Prognosis	What is the likelihood that a patient will develop an illness, or what are the possible health outcomes for the patient with this condition?	Cohort Case-control Case series
Experience or meaning	What are the patient's or health professional's experiences or concerns about this issue?	Qualitative

Systemic error in study design may occur through the method of sampling, by the test used or by encouraging one outcome or answer above others (8). When testing the efficacy of an intervention (e.g. a treatment), a randomised controlled trial (RCT) is the most suitable design to minimise bias. Systematic reviews collect, appraise, report and, in a meta-analysis, combine the evidence from individual studies. Though still susceptible to bias, they are the best study design to inform clinical and policy decisions.

Effect of confounding and bias on study design and bias

Most, if not all, clinical questions seek a relationship between two variables (e.g. A and B). In decision-making, we are interested, if a relationship exists, in the strength and direction of the relationship between an exposure (or intervention) and an outcome, particularly where the relationship is causal (e.g. does smoking [exposure] cause heart disease? [outcome]; does lowering blood pressure [exposure or intervention] reduce the incidence of stroke? [outcome]). Medicine is about improving outcomes. Clinical research is about understanding how exposures or interventions relate to outcomes. Three types of relationships exist between the two – association, correlation and causation (Box 4.5). Establishing causal relationships between exposure and outcome is crucial in evidence-based medicine and governs the choice of study design for the type of clinical or research question.

It is not difficult to demonstrate associations in healthcare. However, the effect of confounding variables makes it more challenging to demonstrate a causal relationship between exposures and outcomes. A confounding variable (confounder) is a factor

Box 4.5 **Relationships between exposure and outcomes in medicine**

- An association between two variables refers to any relationship between the two.
- A correlation refers to a linear relationship between two variables (e.g. as one variable increases, so does the other one).
- A causal relationship between two variables means the presence of the first variable leads to the change in human response observed as the second variable.

other than the one being studied that is associated both with the disease (dependent variable) and with the factor being studied (independent variable). A confounding variable may distort or mask the effects of another variable on the disease in question. For example, we may wish to assess the effects of drinking on the blood pressure of middle-aged women. Unless we account for the confounding effect on blood pressure of smoking in both drinkers and non-drinkers, our results will not have established the true relationship between alcohol consumption and blood pressure in this population. Accounting for confounding variables in research design is vital for ensuring the results of research accurately account for the impact of the variable being studied. Experimental studies help to establish causality. Establishing causality increases the internal validity of the study and increases its wider application in practice.

Advantages and disadvantages of the designs

The RCT is often cited as the 'gold standard' in medical research. This is true but only for certain types of research questions. So, it is the design of choice for assessing the efficacy and effectiveness of a new type of hip replacement. However, an RCT tells us nothing about the experiences, barriers and facilitators for patients recovering from the new surgery. For this, a qualitative study design would be appropriate (Chapter 5). It is essential to understand the strengths and weaknesses of each type of study design, both for our own research and when retrieving a study to answer a clinical question about a patient (Table 4.2).

Randomised controlled trial

An experimental comparison study in which participants are allocated to treatment/intervention or control/placebo groups using a random mechanism (randomisation). Best for studying the effects of an intervention (Figure 4.2).

Non-randomised trials

In this design, participants are allocated to intervention or control groups but in a non-random manner. The allocation may occur because of certain features of the participant or because the participant requests to be in a particular group. An example is a low-cost public campaign in Italy to reduce antibiotic prescribing in upper respiratory tract infection (15). The intervention group was selected non-randomly and exposed to posters, leaflets and advertisements in local media, while the control group in a different region of Italy

Table 4.2 Advantages and disadvantages of different study design.

Design	Type of design	Advantages	Disadvantages
Randomised controlled trial	Experimental	Randomisation leads to unbiased distribution of confounders May help establish causation Well controlled Blinding and concealment more likely	Expensive in time and money Not always feasible or ethical Volunteer or participant bias may exist
Example: Prostate-cancer mortality at 11 years of follow-up. *N Engl J Med* (2012) 366 (11): 981–990. https://doi.org/10.1056/NEJMoa1113135. Erratum in: *N Engl J Med* (2012) 366 (22): 2137. PMID: 22417251; PMCID: PMC6027585.			
Non-randomised control trial	Experimental	Can be used if an RCT is not feasible	Intervention and control groups may not be comparable
Example: A controlled, before-and-after trial of an urban sanitation intervention to reduce enteric infections in children: research protocol for the Maputo Sanitation (MapSan) study, Mozambique. *BMJ Open* (2015) 5 (6): e008215. https://doi.org/10.1136/bmjopen-2015-008215. PMID: 26088809; PMCID: PMC4480002.			
Crossover	Experimental	Better statistical power Participants act as their own controls reducing sample size and variance All subjects receive the intervention at some point Statistical tests assuming randomisation can be used Study can be blinded	Carryover and spillover effects All participants receive the placebo or alternative treatment at some point Washout period is unknown Cannot be used for an intervention with permanents effects (e.g. surgical)
Example: Cluster-randomized crossover trial of chlorhexidine-alcohol versus iodine-alcohol for prevention of surgical-site infection (SKINFECT trial). *BJS Open* (2020) 4 (4): 731–733. https://doi.org/10.1002/bjs5.50285. Epub 2020 Apr 30. PMID: 32352222; PMCID: PMC7397361.			
Case control	Observational	Fewer participants needed than cross-sectional studies Appropriate for very rare disorders or where there is a long interval between exposure and disease	Relies on recall or records to determine exposure – source of potential bias Potential for selection bias
Example: Case-control study of human papillomavirus and oropharyngeal cancer. *N Engl J Med* (2007) 356 (19): 1944–1956. https://doi.org/10.1056/NEJMoa065497. PMID: 17494927.			
Cohort	Observational	Ethically safe Participants can be studied over time Multiple outcomes can be assessed Can be used to assess timing and directionality of events Eligibility criteria and outcome assessment can be standardised Administratively easier and cheaper than RCT	Long timeline until results may not be practical Exposure may be linked to a hidden confounder Blinding is difficult Randomisation not present Large sample sizes and/or long follow-up required for rare conditions
Example: Individual and combined associations between cardiorespiratory fitness and grip strength with common mental disorders: a prospective cohort study in the UK Biobank. *BMC Med* (2020) 18 (1): 303. https://doi.org/10.1186/s12916-020-01782-9. PMID: 33172457; PMCID: PMC7656705.			
Cross-sectional	Observational	Collect a lot of information about a particular situation in time Inexpensive Ethically safe	Requires large sample sizes for accurate results Only valid at the time the study was done Establishes association, not causality Risk of recall bias Confounders may be unequally distributed between groups Group sizes may be unequal
Example: Recent trends in COPD prevalence in Spain: a repeated cross-sectional survey 1997-2007. *Eur Respir J* (2010) 36 (4): 758–765. https://doi.org/10.1183/09031936.00138409. Epub 2009 Dec 8. PMID: 19996189.			

Source: Brown et al. (9), Schröder et al. (10), Aho Glélé et al. (11), D'Souza et al. (12), Kandola et al. (13), Soriano et al. (14).

received no information. The intervention did significantly reduce the rate of antibiotic prescribing. However, it was not clear whether the outcome was due solely to the campaign or other factors (e.g. an outbreak of upper respiratory infections and/or a greater prevalence of smoking in the control group region).

Crossover design

A controlled trial where each study participant has both therapies, for example, is randomised to treatment A first; at the crossover point, they start treatment B. This design is suitable only if the outcome is reversible with time (e.g. symptoms) (Figure 4.3).

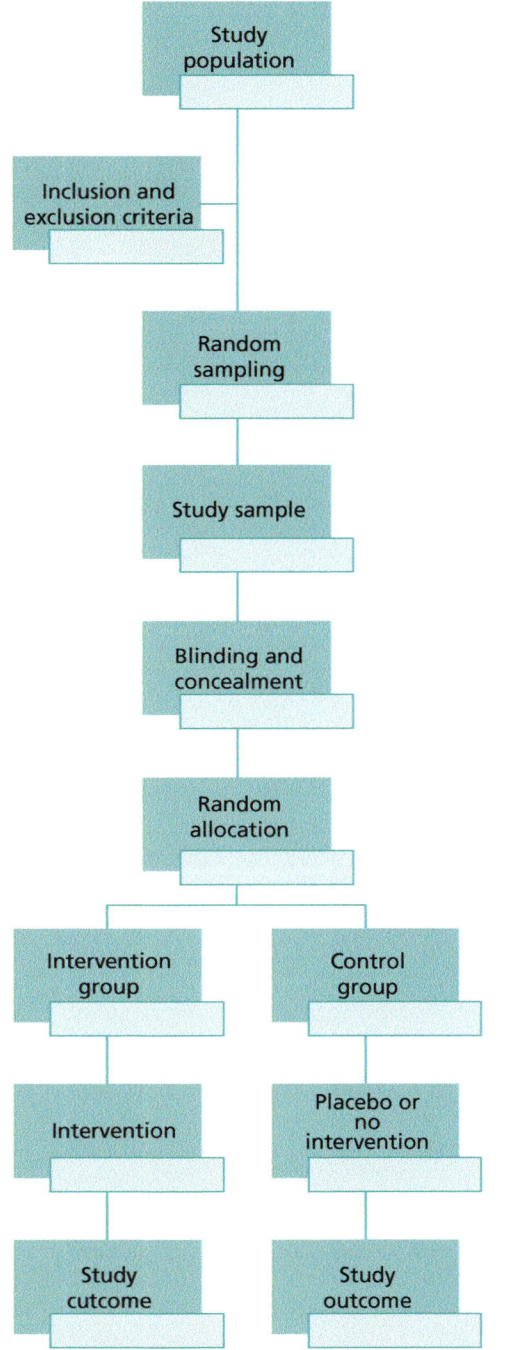

Figure 4.2 Flow chart for the structure of a randomised controlled trial.

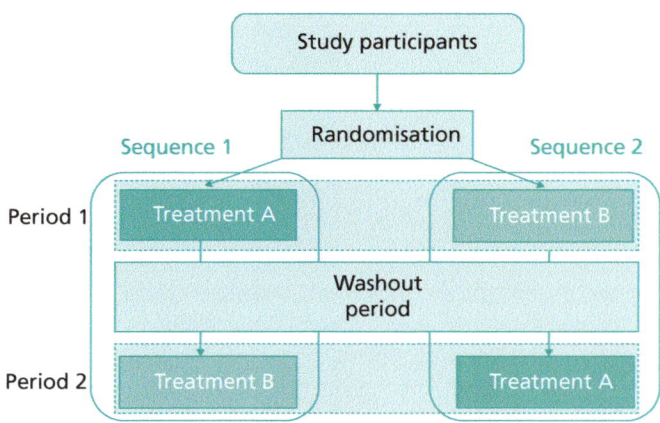

Figure 4.3 Flow chart for design and analysis of a crossover trial. *Source:* Zeng et al. (16)/Springer Nature/CC BY 4.0. This article is licenced under a Creative Commons Attribution 4.0 International License, which permits use, sharing, adaptation, distribution and reproduction in any medium or format, as long as you give appropriate credit to the original author(s) and the source, provide a link to the Creative Commons licence, and indicate if changes were made. The images or other third-party material in this article are included in the article's Creative Commons licence, unless indicated otherwise in a credit line to the material.

Cohort study

Data are obtained from groups who have been exposed, or not exposed, to the new technology or factor of interest (e.g. from databases). No allocation of exposure is made by the researcher. This study is best for studying the effect of predictive risk factors on an outcome (Figure 4.4).

Case-control studies

Patients with a certain outcome or disease and an appropriate group of controls without the outcome or disease are selected (usually with careful consideration of appropriate choice of controls, matching, etc.), and then information is obtained on whether the subjects have been exposed to the factor under investigation (Figure 4.5).

Cross-sectional survey

A study that examines the relationship between disease (or other health-related characteristics) and other variables of interest as they exist in a defined population at one particular time (i.e. exposure and outcomes are both measured at the same time). This study is best for quantifying the prevalence of a disease or risk factor and for quantifying the accuracy of a diagnostic test (Figure 4.6).

Designing and planning a study

Review of literature

Once the question is formulated, the literature on the topic should be comprehensively reviewed. This ensures familiarity with information published previously on the topic. It may also retrieve previously published research of relevance to the new research question.

Formulating hypotheses

Since particularly experimental studies will wish to determine the effect of an intervention, a hypothesis should be defined at the outset. A hypothesis is a proposed explanation for the outcome observed in the experiment (e.g. clinical trial). Hypotheses should be defined in terms that are measurable and easily understood. Any assumptions about the study, population, observed or experimental intervention should be made explicit. The hypothesis is described in two ways:

- The null hypothesis which states there is no difference in the outcome of interest (e.g. mortality rate) between the two groups.
- The alternative hypothesis states there is a difference in the outcomes between the two groups. This difference may be in either direction (two-tailed) or in the direction of the effect (one-tailed). Both hypotheses will be analysed in the results stage of the study (Chapter 6).

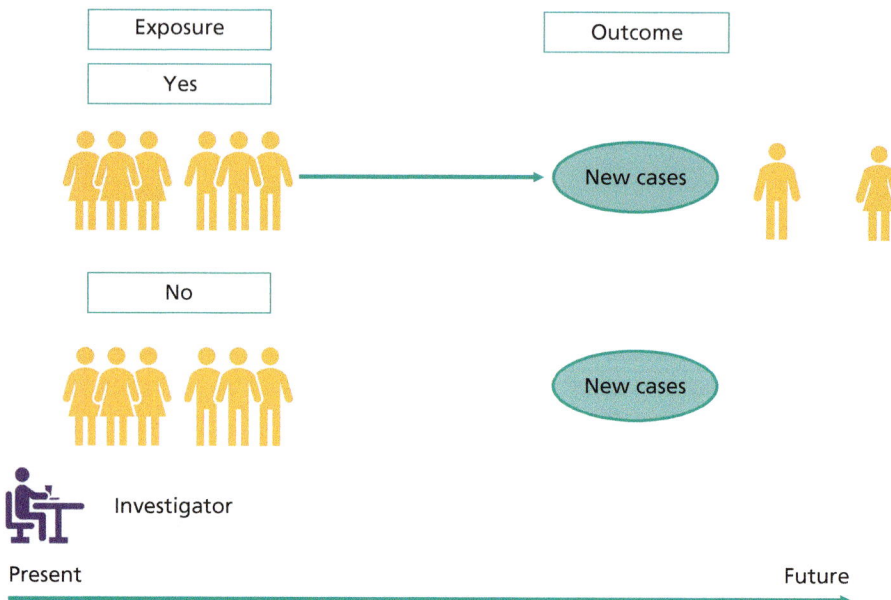

Figure 4.4 Design of a prospective cohort study.

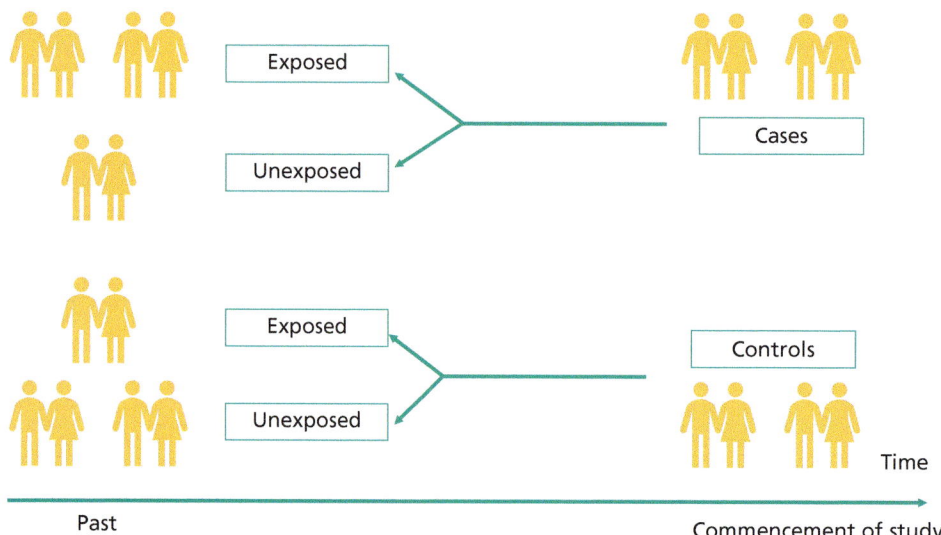

Figure 4.5 Case-control study design.

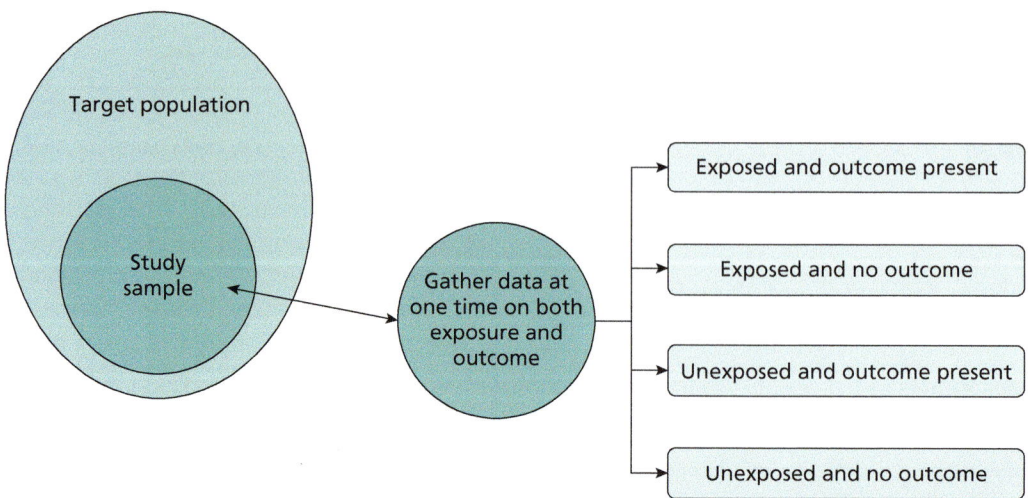

Figure 4.6 Cross-sectional study design. *Source:* Wang and Cheng (17)/with permission of Elsevier.

Specification of needed data

The investigators should determine the kind of data required to test the hypothesis. Each part of the hypothesis should be scrutinised for the specific data to be obtained to test it adequately.

Methods and techniques to yield data needed

Methods to obtain the required data should be determined. What kinds of samples are necessary? A finding obtained from a sample may be generalised only when the individuals studied constitute a random or representative sample of the wider population. Random (or representative) sampling requires that every member of the population or group has an equal probability of being drawn in the sample, and second, each member drawn in the sample be studied or in some way accounted for in the study protocol and analysis. For each individual selection, the probability for each person of being selected must be constant.

A frequent question concerns the size of the sample needed. The required sample size is estimated in terms of the complexity of the analyses to be made, the heterogeneity of the population regarding the characteristics to be studied, the degree of precision of findings required and the kinds of statistical measures to be used. Factors include the expected effect size (i.e. the difference between the groups, the standard deviation of the population for continuous data, the desired power of the study to detect the hypothesised effect and the level of significance sought).

Planning the analysis

Setting up blank or dummy tables showing which data are to be obtained and how they may be related to other data and in what manner indicate any gaps in the data and may occasionally show that more data are being sought than actually required. Indicating the kinds of statistical calculations envisaged helps to determine the minimum sample size needed. Analysis planning may reveal if the form in which the data are to be collected will facilitate the statistical analysis.

Pretesting study design and data collection

The instruments can be pretested on a small but representative sample of the population (pilot study). By this stage, up to 90% of the time spent on the study will have been spent on planning the data collection and analysis.

Analysis and interpretation of data

The analysis plan developed at the outset is applied to the collected data. The data is summarised. Where hypotheses have been stated clearly, interpretations of data are always clearer than where hypotheses are vaguely stated or not stated at all. In the latter situation, the investigators are required to rationalise the data after the fact, a situation that is prone to bias. An important obligation of the researcher is communicating their methods and findings to colleagues clearly to facilitate further research so others can build further on their results and to enable wider implementation of findings.

Misconceptions

Research should be based on rational, systematic planning. The person who can develop a sound plan will rarely have trouble communicating its aims or results. The person who has difficulty communicating a good plan probably does not have one.

A second misconception is that inadequate research designs can be made acceptable by labelling them 'exploratory'. Investigation of previously unresearched fields often involves exploration of imperfectly defined hypotheses or incompletely developed methods. However, the exploratory researcher is still obliged ethically and professionally to observe the principles of sound research design to the maximum extent possible and to account when, how and why this has not been possible.

A third misconception is that basic research, in which research is an end, is good, and that applied research, in which research is a means to an end, is poor. It is both possible and imperative to develop sound research designs in applied research, and it is not unusual to encounter poor design in basic research.

What is a clinical trial?

Clinical trials are the gold standard for evaluation of healthcare interventions (18). A research project which compares two or more treatments in patients with a particular condition or at risk of a condition can help generate high-quality evidence about which is the more effective treatment or preventative strategy (18). The treatment being investigated in a clinical trial can be a medicinal product, a procedure, a device or other type of therapeutic intervention. Clinical trials are an essential part of evidence-based practice. They can guide treatment decisions for both healthcare professionals and patients. Clinical trials are an important part of the pathways by which new medicinal products can obtain a licence from the Medicine and Healthcare products Regulatory Agency (MHRA) and become available for use as new treatments.

A clinical trial is appropriate when there is uncertainty about which treatment options or preventive strategies are most effective. A trial seeks to confirm an intervention is safe as well as effective. Trials should be designed with the aim of contributing to future decision-making. The trial team may involve clinicians, researchers, statisticians and health economists. Ethical approval will be required, and the investigators will need to demonstrate training in research integrity and the legal aspects of conducting trials.

It is easier to demonstrate correlation than causation. The impact of the intervention must be isolated from other effects by controlling for potential biases, confounding factors and by minimising variation between groups.

Planning a clinical trial

It is important to establish the need for a new trial. Every trial begins by defining the fundamental question being asked. An initially vague concept must be developed into an answerable and quantifiable hypothesis. Planning can be considered as two phases: (i) conceptual and (ii) implementation (Figure 4.7) (19).

Conceptual phase

The planning process itself, including the protocol, permissions and ethical approval, can take up to a year. The investigators and funders should undertake a systematic review of the existing research (18).

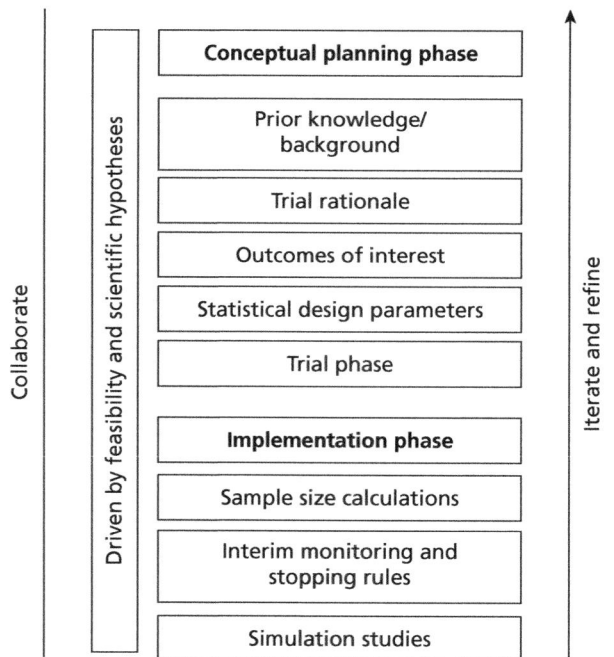

Figure 4.7 Principles for conceptual planning and implementation stages of clinical trials. *Source:* Duong et al. (20) with permission of Elsevier.

This may answer the original research question. If not, the review establishes the need for the trial and contributes to its design. The time for the trial itself will depend on the sample size, the ease with which participants are recruited and the period of follow-up required to observe the intervention effects in each participant.

Important steps in trial design include minimising variation between intervention and control groups, effective randomisation and stratification of the sample groups, determining blinding procedures, use of placebos, selection of the population and a sample within it and the selection of robust endpoints to determine the outcome of the trial.

Once made, it is difficult to rectify mistakes in trial design. A statistician should be involved at an early stage. This ensures the sample size calculation is accurate. Equally important is ensuring the statistical hypothesis aligns with the study objectives and that statistical analyses are applied correctly (19). Bespoke trial designs may be required for rare diseases (21). Trial outcomes should be determined at an early stage. These may be either health- or treatment-related (Box 4.6).

It is common to have one or two primary outcomes and one or two secondary outcomes (19). Primary outcomes are related to the mechanism of action of the intervention, clinically meaningful, relevant to the patient, clearly defined and measurable (19).

Single-arm trials versus randomisation

In single-arm studies, all patients receive the same intervention. The control is provided by a historical group. This approach does introduce bias as the single arm and historical control may not be from the same population and, in any event, have received the intervention under different conditions. A randomised design is preferable when possible.

Box 4.6 Clinical trial outcomes

Health-related
- Quality of life
- Symptoms
- Adverse events
- Patient-reported outcomes

Treatment-related
- Safety or efficacy of the intervention
- Tumour shrinkage
- Haematological outcomes
- Intermediate or surrogate outcomes
- Time to event outcomes
  - Overall survival
  - Progression-free survival
- Surgical outcomes

Source: Duong et al.(20) with permission of Elsevier.

Randomisation (19)

Randomisation aims to create two or more groups similar in respect to all factors which might affect the outcome except for the intervention. It is an attempt to deal with confounding variables within a population. The commonest design is an intervention arm and a control arm (which receives either standard care or a placebo). Randomisation is often combined with other measures to reduce bias, including blinding and allocation concealment. Randomisation may be balanced where groups are of equal size or unbalanced where the numbers in each group are unequal. Even after following randomisation, differences may remain between groups. These variables may confound the analysis and include gender, age and factors relevant to the study outcomes. Stratification addresses this with participants allocated to groups according to the relevant factors and then randomised within each stratum.

Blinding and concealment

Randomisation reduces the effects of selection bias and confounding variables. Allocation of participants to intervention and control groups should be a random sequence. The allocation should be concealed (concealment) from those involved in the trial. This is referred to as blinding (or 'masking') and means withholding information having the potential to influence the results from one or more parties to those involved in the research study. In single blinding, the patient does not know to which group they have been allocated; in double blinding, neither patient nor investigator knows the allocation, while in triple blinding, the allocation is withheld also from those analysing the study data. Without this, patients and investigators have been known to change allocations with the result that groups become less equivalent.

Pilot study

A pilot study establishes the potential difficulties of conducting the proposed trial. It is also helpful in calculating the required sample size. Difficulty in establishing robust outcomes for a trial or if the mechanism of a proposed intervention (e.g. treatment) has not been established, it may be more appropriate to conduct an observational study (18).

Trial phase

The trial phase occurs from preclinical use of the intervention to post-marketing surveillance. Early phases include pilot study, phase I and II, single arm and proof of concept. Later phases include randomised phase II, II/III and phase III trials. Phase II trials evaluate the safety and efficacy of an intervention and whether to proceed to phase III. Given the importance of safely moving from a phase II trial to larger-scale use in a phase III trial, the endpoints used in phase II should mirror strongly those used in phase III (19).

Common pitfalls in clinical trials

Whilst working in an experienced Clinical Trials Unit (CTU) helps to reduce the risk of problems, nonetheless problems exist and include underestimating the time to develop the protocol and securing permissions including ethical approval. Recruitment needs to be timely to ensure the trial can proceed within the desired time frame. There should be mechanisms for monitoring adverse events. These may require review by the ethics committee and an independent data monitoring committee to ensure participants are not being harmed by the intervention. A trial may need to be terminated early if harm is occurring to either the intervention or control group. For example, in the SPRINT study comparing intense and standard treatment for hypertension, the trial was stopped early after participants in the intensive treatment group were found to have a 25% lower risk from major cardiovascular events and a 27% lower relative risk from any cause compared to those in the standard treatment group (7).

Evidence synthesis

One of the great achievements of evidence-based healthcare is evidence synthesis. This is exemplified most significantly by the systematic review. In Chapter 1, we highlighted the role of the Cochrane Collaboration in promoting and publishing systematic reviews. Though Cochrane has led the way, systematic reviews are now published across many journals. For the researcher, systematic reviews are a starting point for new studies and trials; for the frontline clinician, a comprehensive summary of evidence to facilitate decision-making; and for the policymaker, an important resource in the implementation of research findings.

What is evidence synthesis? (22)

This methodology has been applied not only in healthcare but also in education, law, international development and the environment. Evidence synthesis involves interpretation of all the individual studies on a given subject. The purpose is to provide a rigorous and transparent 'evidence base' which can be utilised for translation of research into practice and policy. The process requires the use of explicit and transparent methodology. Reporting should include how studies were retrieved, selected, appraised and analysed. The strength of the evidence should be stated in making any recommendation. Though the systematic review is the best known and most utilised methodology, many others exist (Box 4.7).

Prior to systematic reviews, evidence synthesis was usually via literature or narrative reviews. However, these are prone to bias

Box 4.7 **Evidence synthesis methodologies**

- Evidence maps
- Literature reviews
- Living reviews
- Mixed method reviews
- Qualitative evidence reviews
- Rapid reviews
- Realist synthesis
- Scoping reviews
- Systematic reviews
- Umbrella reviews

Source: Munn et al. (23)/Springer Nature/CC BY 4.0.

due to inadequate searching, subjective topic choice and an unstructured appraisal. The methodology is not standardised across all literature reviews.

Systematic reviews

A systematic review is a synthesis of literature which is focused on a well-formulated research question. The review aims to identify and synthesise all research on a topic, published and unpublished. It should be conducted in an unbiased and reproducible way. Where studies included in the review contain statistical information, this may also be synthesised to draw inferences about much larger samples or populations than would be possible from single studies. The systematic review is conducted using a protocol developed before the initial evidence search is undertaken. Reasons for conducting a systematic review include retrieving all available evidence, confirming the scope of current practice in an area and any variations, identifying areas for future research and producing conclusions and statements to guide decision-making. Systematic reviews are undertaken across a range of domains (Table 4.3) (23). Though domains and research questions vary between reviews, they all follow the same basic structure (Figure 4.8).

Registration and reporting of results

It is now best practice that all research be registered in a publicly accessible database. In the case of clinical trials, it is a condition for ethical approval. All outcomes to be measured should be pre-specified at registration. The International Committee of Medical Journal Editors (ICMJE) will only consider trials for publication if they are registered appropriately. A study registered on a public database must report its results within one year of the completion of the study or six months for paediatric research. Publicly accessible registries include ClinicalTrials.gov, ISRCTN and EduraCT. Registration of trials and results prevents selective publication and reporting of results. This reduces duplication of research and ensures the public is aware of ongoing or planned research.

Table 4.3 What type of systematic review should I conduct?

Review type	Aim	Question format
Effectiveness	To evaluate the effectiveness of a treatment/practice in terms of its impact on outcomes	Population, intervention, comparator/s, outcomes (PICO)
Experiential (qualitative)	To investigate the meaning of a particular phenomenon	Population, phenomena of interest, context (PICo)
Cost/economic evaluation	To determine the costs of a particular treatment or strategy, particularly in terms of cost effectiveness or benefit	Population, intervention, comparator/s, outcomes, context (PICOC)
Prevalence and/or incidence	To determine the prevalence and/or incidence of a certain condition	Condition, context, population (CoCoPop)
Diagnostic test accuracy	To determine how well a diagnostic test works in terms of its sensitivity and specificity for a particular diagnosis	Population, index test, reference test, diagnosis of interest (PIRD)
Aetiology and/or risk	To determine the association between particular exposures/risk factors and outcomes	Population, exposure, outcome (PEO)
Expert opinion/policy	To review and synthesise current expert opinion, text or policy on a certain phenomena	Population, intervention or phenomena of interest, context (PICo)
Psychometric	To evaluate the psychometric properties of a certain test, normally to determine the reliability and validity of a particular test or assessment	Construct of interest or the name of the measurement instrument(s), population, type of measurement, measurement properties
Prognostic	To determine the overall prognosis for a condition, the link between specific prognostic factors and outcome and/or prognostic/prediction models and prognostic tests	Population, prognostic factors (or models of interest), outcome (PFO)
Methodology	To examine and investigate current research methods and potentially their impact on research quality	Types of studies, types of data, types of methods, outcomes (SDMO)

Changes made to original table: Column 4 containing example questions has been removed
Open Access This article is distributed under the terms of the Creative Commons Attribution 4.0 International License (http://creativecommons.org/licenses/by/4.0/), which permits unrestricted use, distribution, and reproduction in any medium, provided you give appropriate credit to the original author(s) and the source, provide a link to the Creative Commons license, and indicate if changes were made.
Source: Munn et al. (23).

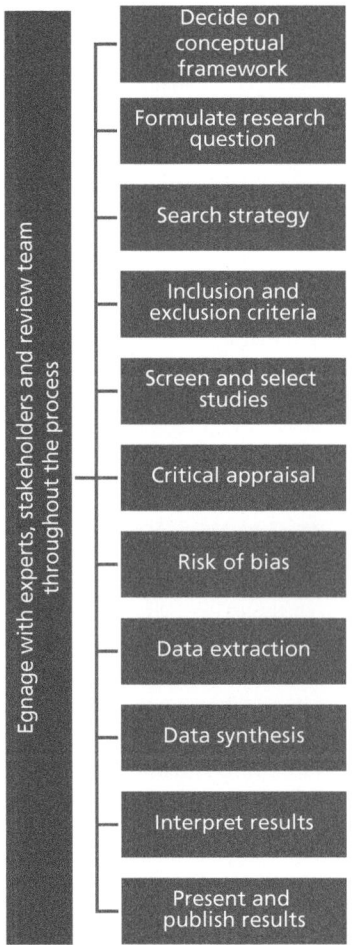

Figure 4.8 Steps in conducting a systematic review.

Table 4.4 Summary of reporting guidelines for each main study design.

Randomised trials	CONSORT	Extensions
Observational studies	STROBE	Extensions
Systematic reviews	PRISMA	Extensions
Study protocols	SPIRIT	PRISMA-P
Diagnostic/prognostic studies	STARD	TRIPOD
Case reports	CARE	Extensions
Clinical practice guidelines	AGREE	RIGHT
Qualitative research	SRQR	COREQ
Quality improvement studies	SQUIRE	Extensions
Economic evaluations	CHEERS	Extensions

Source: Enhancing the QUAlity and Transparency Of health Research, https://www.equator-network.org/, last accessed on September 17, 2024/ Equator-network.

Reporting guidelines

A reporting guideline is:

'a checklist, flow diagram or structured text to guide authors in reporting a specific type of research, developed using explicit methodology' (Equator Network).

Guidelines are collated and made available at the UK EQUATOR Centre at http://equator-network.org (Table 4.4). A guideline exists for each type of study and will have its own website with further information. Each guideline provides a list of items which should be reported. The guidelines are intended to ensure the study is understandable by the general reader, can be replicated by another researcher, can facilitate clinical decision-making and is suitable for inclusion in a systematic review.

References

1 Rosenstock, I.M. and Hochbaum, G.M. (2010). Some principles of research design in public health 1961. *Am J Public Health* 100 (10): 1861–1863.

2 Grimes, D.A. and Schulz, K.F. (2002). An overview of clinical research: the lay of the land. *Lancet* 359 (9300): 57–61.

3 Yuguero, O., Marsal, J.R., Buti, M. et al. (2017). Descriptive study of association between quality of care and empathy and burnout in primary care. *BMC Med Ethics* 18 (1): 54.

4 Ranganathan, P. and Aggarwal, R. (2019). Study designs: part 3 – analytical observational studies. *Perspect Clin Res* 10 (2): 91–94.

5 Viljakainen, H.T., Korhonen, T., Hytinantti, T. et al. (2011). Maternal vitamin D status affects bone growth in early childhood – a prospective cohort study. *Osteoporos Int* 22 (3): 883–891.

6 Bhide, A., Shah, P.S., and Acharya, G. (2018). A simplified guide to randomized controlled trials. *Acta Obstet Gynecol Scand* 97 (4): 380–387.

7 Wright, J.T. Jr., Williamson, J.D., Whelton, P.K. et al. (2015). A randomized trial of intensive versus standard blood-pressure control. *N Engl J Med* 373 (22): 2103–2116.

8 Pannucci, C.J. and Wilkins, E.G. (2010). Identifying and avoiding bias in research. *Plast Reconstr Surg* 126 (2): 619–625.

9 Brown, J., Cumming, O., Bartram, J. et al. (2015). A controlled, before-and-after trial of an urban sanitation intervention to reduce enteric infections in children: research protocol for the Maputo Sanitation (MapSan) study, Mozambique. *BMJ Open* 5 (6): e008215.

10 Schröder, F.H., Hugosson, J., Roobol, M.J. et al. (2012). Prostate-cancer mortality at 11 years of follow-up. *N Engl J Med* 366 (11): 981–990.

11 Aho Glélé, L.S., Ortega-Deballon, P., Guilloteau, A. et al. (2020). Cluster-randomized crossover trial of chlorhexidine-alcohol versus iodine-alcohol for prevention of surgical-site infection (SKINFECT trial). *BJS Open* 4 (4): 731–733.

12 D'Souza, G., Kreimer, A.R., Viscidi, R. et al. (2007). Case-control study of human papillomavirus and oropharyngeal cancer. *N Engl J Med* 356 (19): 1944–1956.

13 Kandola, A.A., Osborn, D.P.J., Stubbs, B. et al. (2020). Individual and combined associations between cardiorespiratory fitness and grip strength with common mental disorders: a prospective cohort study in the UK Biobank. *BMC Med* 18 (1): 303.

14 Soriano, J.B., Ancochea, J., Miravitlles, M. et al. (2010). Recent trends in COPD prevalence in Spain: a repeated cross-sectional survey 1997–2007. *Eur Respir J* 36 (4): 758–765.

15 Sedgwick, P. (2014). What is a non-randomised controlled trial? *BMJ* 348: g4115.

16 Zeng, L., Qureshi, R., Viswanathan, S. et al. (2020). Registration of phase 3 crossover trials on ClinicalTrials.gov. *Trials* 21 (1): 613. https://doi.org/10.1186/s13063-020-04545-2.

17 Wang, X. and Cheng, Z. (2020) Cross-sectional *studies*: strengths, weaknesses, and recommendations. Chest 158(1S): S65–S71. doi: 10.1016/j.chest.2020.03.012. PMID: 32658654.

18 Research NIfHaC (2019). *Clinical Trials Guide*. Leeds: NIHR.

19 An, M.W., Duong, Q., Le-Rademacher, J., and Mandrekar, S.J. (2020). Principles of good clinical trial design. *J Thorac Oncol* 15 (8): 1277–1280.

20 Duong, Q., Le-Rademacher, J., Mandrekar, S.J. (2020) Principles of good clinical trial design. *J Thorac Oncol* 15(8):1277–1280. doi: 10.1016/j.jtho.2020.05.005. PMID: 32417343; PMCID: PMC7390662.

21 Gupta, S., Faughnan, M.E., Tomlinson, G.A., and Bayoumi, A.M. (2011). A framework for applying unfamiliar trial designs in studies of rare diseases. *J Clin Epidemiol* 64 (10): 1085–1094.

22 Evidence Synthesis International (2020). What is evidence synthesis? https://evidencesynthesis.org/what-is-evidence-synthesis/.

23 Munn, Z., Stern, C., Aromataris, E. et al. (2018). What kind of systematic review should I conduct? A proposed typology and guidance for systematic reviewers in the medical and health sciences. *BMC Med Res Methodol* 18 (1): 5.

Further reading

Centre for Evidence-Based Medicine. University of Oxford. https://www.cebm.ox.ac.uk/resources/ebm-tools/study-designs.

CHAPTER 5

Qualitative Research

John Frain

Division of Medical Sciences and Graduate Entry Medicine, University of Nottingham, Nottingham, UK

OVERVIEW

- Different research questions require different study designs.
- Qualitative research is important in discovering the lived experience of patients in relation to health, experience of symptoms, diagnosis, treatment and living with disease.
- Qualitative research bridges the gap between a patient's and practitioner's practical experience.
- It facilitates transfer of knowledge into practice.
- Qualitative and quantitative can be combined to produce a mixed-methods study design.

Introduction

Through emphasis on quantitative data and biostatistics, clinical epidemiology underpins evidence-based medicine (EBM). Its concepts facilitate decisions about disease risk, diagnosis, treatment and prognosis. Quantitative methods use numerical data. Statistical analysis of this numerical data enables the research to draw inferences about the phenomenon studied (Chapter 6). By contrast, qualitative research with an emphasis on personal observation, reflection and judgement can seem unscientific and subjective. Those new to EBM and research can initially regard small samples and a lack of numbers and statistical tests as evidence of poor research. In fact, qualitative research investigates practitioners and patients' attitudes, beliefs and preferences and how evidence is turned into practice (1). EBM is not simply the application of the results of randomised controlled trials (RCTs). Exploration also needs to be made of the limitations of trials and and of the barriers for patients and practitioners. (Box 5.1). The differences between quantitative and qualitative research are shown in Table 5.1 (2).

'Qualitative research involves broadly stated questions about human experiences and realities, studied through sustained contact with the individual in their natural environments and producing rich, descriptive data that will help us understand those individual's experiences' (3). Examples of qualitative research questions in healthcare include:

- What is the experience of medical students in developing clinical reasoning?
- Why are healthcare staff experiencing increased rates of burnout?
- How do diabetic patients develop the self-confidence to give their own insulin injections?
- Why do LGBTQ+ patients have anxieties about accessing healthcare in the United Kingdom?
- In women with coronary heart disease, what is their experience of receiving the diagnosis?
- Is dietary advice given by the National Health Service (NHS) tailored to the lived experience of patients of South Asian ethnicity?

All the aforementioned questions are concerned with people's experience and the way they understand things. Answering them requires exploring patterns and reasons for behaviour. Qualitative research draws on approaches in sociology, psychology and anthropology. There are different methodologies within the concepts of qualitative research. They all share basic orientations (Box 5.2) (1). The results of qualitative research facilitate the development of future health interventions and explanatory health models (2). They also help identify research questions for future quantitative studies. Qualitative research did not initially fall into the scope of evidence-based healthcare. Currently, perspectives of the patient and clinician are required alongside the quantitative evaluation of a new therapy.

Understanding the orientations of both patients and practitioners can enable the design of better quantitative research with more emphasis on how results will be translated into real-world practice. The focus of quantitative research is often around interactions either person to person or, for example, with environments, treatments, devices or treatment regimens. The pragmatic RCT is an example of combining quantitative and qualitative approaches to assess the effectiveness of an intervention (4).

Box 5.1 **Example of a qualitative research in healthcare**

This study examined the experiences of 22 US health workers during the first wave of the Covid-19 pandemic. Fourteen were female and three from a racial or ethnic minority population. Semi-structured interviews were conducted and transcribed using a social-ecological model. Interviews were analysed using thematic analysis to generate major themes and subthemes. Major themes identified included (i) institutions, infrastructure and the pandemic; (ii) working under fire; (iii) the political becomes personal; and (iv) hope. Phenomena at personal, interpersonal, community, organisational and societal levels affected health workers' experiences and suggested mechanisms by which impacts on health workers' physical and mental health could be mitigated.

Source: Adapted from Goff et al. (19).

Box 5.2 **Basis orientations of qualitative methods**

- Naturalism – what is the everyday context in which healthcare takes place?
- Interpretation – what is the meaning of symptoms and diagnoses experienced by patients and practitioners?
- Process – do the meanings of these experiences change over time?
- Interaction – how does the communication between patients and practitioners affect the healthcare experience?
- Relativism – is the 'reality' experienced by patients the same or different from that of practitioners?

Source: Adapted from Green and Britten (1).

Table 5.1 Differences between quantitative and qualitative research.

Areas	Quantitative research	Qualitative research
Goal	Test and confirm hypotheses	Explore and understand phenomena
Data collection methods	Highly structured questionnaires, inventories, tests and scales	Interviews, observations and focus group discussions
Design	Pre-planned, protocol driven and rigid design	Flexible and emergent design
Reasoning	Deductive – hypothesis testing	Primarily inductive by the researcher to develop the theory
Focus	Outcomes, prediction of the causal relationships and numbers	Quality – features of the process, rather than outcomes or products
Sampling	Largely random sampling methods	Purposive sampling methods
Sample size determination	Involves a priori sample size calculation	Collect data until data saturation is achieved
Sample size	Relatively large	Small sample size but studied in-depth
Data analysis	Analysis of variables using statistics or mathematical methods	Case based and uses non-statistical description or interpretation

Source: Adapted from Renjith V, Yesodharan R, Noronha JA, Ladd E, George A. Qualitative Methods in Health Care Research. Int J Prev Med. 2021;12:20.

The qualitative research question

As in quantitative research, the initial question is important in developing the study protocol, selecting the design and developing the data collection and methods of analysis. Qualitative questions tend to be exploratory and open-ended (2). There are two parts – a main question and related subquestions, usually no more than five to seven (2). The PCO format is used to structure the question (Box 5.3).

Data in qualitative research

Instead of numbers, qualitative data can be words, images, documents or audio recordings. These are interpreted by the researcher. Data may be collected as an end in itself, or it may be

Box 5.3 **Example of a qualitative research question using the PCO format**

The PCO format is commonly used in qualitative research where P is the population under study, C is the context of exploration and O is the outcome of interest. So for the question:
 'What is the experience of graduate entry medical students in developing early clinical reasoning during the preclinical phase of their training?'
 P is graduate entry medical students.
 C is the preclinical phase of training.
 O is the students' experiences of developing early clinical reasoning.

Source: Adapted from Butler et al. (20).

Box 5.4 **Trustworthiness in qualitative research**

- Transferable – the concepts presented by the data interpretation are applicable in both the study setting and the wider community.
- Credibility – the account of the research is believable in terms of the participant's stories and the researcher's interpretations.
- Reflexivity – does the researcher display reflection and explanation of their own impact on the project?
- Transparency – is the planning, rationale for decision-making and delivery of the study, the data analysis and presentation of results explicit and clear?

Source: Adapted from Williams et al. (5).

used to generate a new theory or model to be used as the basis for further research. Both outcomes reflect the researcher's interpretation. This sounds far more subjective than the 'objectivity' of numbers-based quantitative research, though the latter still depends on human interpretation. Rather than the objectivity, the qualitative researcher aims for 'trustworthiness' in their study results (Box 5.4) (5).

Qualitative study designs

Qualitative research covers several study designs. These are ethnography, grounded theory, phenomenology, case study and narrative analysis. Key characteristics of qualitative methodology are summarised in Box 5.5.

Ethnography (6)

In healthcare, ethnography explores the behaviours, interactions and links of a 'culture-sharing group'. 'Culture sharing group' describes any group of people who share common meanings, customs or experiences (e.g. healthcare students, sports or music fans and members of a religious community). The focus is usually on the context or culture of the group. Data collection is via observation, interviews, audiovisual and written records. The written report contains the views of the participants (emic perspectives) and the researchers' views of the culture (etic perspectives).

Grounded theory (6)

Grounded theory is the generation of explanations or theories in the context of the reality (the grounding) of the participants' experience. Data collection is through recording and analysis of interviews with participants until data saturation is reached (Box 5.6).

Data analysis occurs in a three-step process – 'open coding', 'axial coding' and 'selective coding'. Open coding involves creation of a broad range of categories of terms within the data. Axial coding identifies connections between the open codes. Selective coding then connects the axial codes to formulate a theory to explain the study question. Quotes from participants are used to support the findings. 'The value of the grounded theory lies not only in its ability to generate a theory but also to ground that theory in the data' (7).

Phenomenology (6)

Phenomenology is the discovery of the essence of an individual's experience and to distil this into a central meaning of how a phenomenon is experienced by a person or group. In healthcare,

---

Box 5.6 **What is data saturation?**

Data saturation is the point in a qualitative study where the data collection is no longer identifying new information. The concept was developed in 1967 in relation to grounded theory research. The concept is important for sample size calculation. A review of 23 studies found that, relative to quantitative methods, smaller samples achieve data saturation in qualitative methodology. For interviews, 9–17 participants or 4–8 focus group discussions were sufficient. However, this applied more to homogenous study populations and narrowly defined study objectives. Multi-country research, meta-themes and 'code meaning' saturation require larger samples.

Source: Adapted from Hennink and Kaiser (21).

---

phenomenological studies often examine life transitions (e.g. newly qualified doctors beginning clinical practice; patients adjusting to a diagnosis of cancer; medical students' assimilation of professional values during training). Data is collected usually by interviews, focus groups, documents and observation may also be involved.

Data analysis involves identification of significant meanings and answering, 'What was experienced? How was it experienced? And what does this mean for the person?' Descriptive phenomenology concerns describing the essential features and structures of a phenomenon. Interpretive phenomenology concentrates instead on the meaning and significance of the experiences.

Case study research (6)

This focuses on the description and in-depth analysis of the case(s). Analysis involves studying an event, an activity or an illness. Data collection is via observation, one-to-one interviews, artefacts and documents. Analysis is done through description of the case. From this themes and cross-themes are identified. The written report will include a detailed description of one or more cases.

Narrative research

This is 'story telling' of an individual life. Data is collected as a 'story' through interviews, field notes and documents. It is often reported as in the first person.

Historical research

'Systematic collection, critical evaluation, and interpretation of historical evidence. Data is usually collected from primary and secondary sources' (1).

Conducting a qualitative research study

In this section, we will illustrate some of the concepts from a qualitative study of facilitators and barriers to prevention of non-communicable diseases in Pakistan (Box 5.7).

Box 5.5 **Key characteristics of qualitative research**

- Flexibility – the design can be adjusted to emerging themes as the data is collected.
- Data collection – various methods can be incorporated into the design, including one-to-one interviews, focus groups and diaries.
- Focus is on an individual or group experience or in a social setting.
- Emphasis is on understanding the whole rather than only a part of the phenomenon under study.
- The researcher is intensely involved in the collection of data.
- Ongoing analysis of the data as the study proceeds enables further data collection and theory development.
- A model is developed from the data as it emerges, as opposed to quantitative research, where a hypothesis is proposed and then data is collected to confirm or refute it.

Source: Offredy (8)/John Wiley & Sons.

Sampling (8)

In contrast to quantitative studies, sampling is non-random and non-probability. There are several techniques. The most used techniques are convenience, purposive, snowball and intensity sampling.

Convenience sampling
Participants are invited to join the study based on their accessibility, geographical proximity, ease, speed and low cost. This sampling method may result in issues with representation and inclusion in the study.

Purposive sampling
Subjects are selective from an already identified population. Choosing information-rich cases is key to determining the power and logic of purposive sampling.

Snowball sampling
Also known as 'chain referral sampling' or 'network sampling.' The sample starts with a few initial participants. The researcher relies on these early participants to identify additional participants. It is useful where the researcher wishes to identify a marginalised group or community and in other studies where participants may be difficult to identify. Respondent-driven sampling is a variant of snowball sampling where respondents are selected from a social network of existing members of the sample.

Intensity sampling
The process of identifying data- or information-rich sources is known as intensity sampling. The researcher undertakes preliminary evaluation of the topic and variation within the group to be studied. Once variation has been identified (extreme, average and intense), the researcher identifies intense cases within the sample population.

Determining the sample size

Qualitative research sample sizes are smaller than quantitative studies. In the latter, large samples are required to enable the calculation of statistically significant information. In qualitative research, data collection goes deep into individuals' experiences rather than widely across the characteristics of populations. A key conception in qualitative sampling is data saturation.

Data saturation (or point of redundancy) is the stage at which the researcher no longer hears or observes any new information. At this point, the researcher has captured all information about the topic under study. When no further or new information is being captured, data collection can be stopped. In the study in Box 5.7, a purposive sample was chosen from a population of over 18 years of age with established non-communicable disease.

Data collection

A variety of methods can be used to collect data in qualitative studies. The most commonly used are focus groups, one-to-one in-depth interviews and participant observation (Table 5.2). Other methods in healthcare are narrative life history, document analysis, audio and video footage, text analysis and simple observation.

Focus groups (8)
Focus groups facilitate the collection of data on a topic from several individuals in the study group. This includes capturing the range of perspectives regarding the topic of study. Given the practicalities of time and enabling people to speak, the size of a focus group is usually between 6 and 12. Focus groups may be homogeneous or heterogeneous, depending on the group. In our example study, an initial sample of 16–20 participants was sought. The process was iterative. Data saturation was achieved with 30 participants who were interviewed in four separate groups each lasting 60–90 minutes (10).

One-to-one interviews
These enable the in-depth exploration of a single participant's experience, including personal history, lived experiences, perceptions and views. They are useful in the study of personal or sensitive subjects. Interviews may be structured, unstructured or semi-structured in terms of using predetermined questions.

Interview topic guide

Even in unstructured interviews, it is helpful for the researcher to have an initial list of questions. This helps initiate the conversation with the researcher and then allows the participant to lead the discussion (Box 5.8).

Table 5.2 Advantages and disadvantages of methods of data collection in qualitative research.

Method	Advantages	Disadvantages
Focus group	• Efficient collection from multiple people • Richer data results from participant interaction • Safe space if participants are comfortable with one another	• Difficult to coordinate a convenient time and place • If figures of authority are present (i.e. senior staff), some participants may be inhibited from speaking openly • Quieter people may not have a chance to speak • Difficult to conduct remotely
Interviews	• Facilitates discussion of sensitive or difficult topics • Rich data on individual, personal experiences • More flexible to arrange	• Data collection takes longer than focus groups • Expensive and time-consuming to transcribe and analyse
Observations	• Helpful to observe how things happen in real life; not based on opinion • Reduces the influence of the researcher on data interpretation	• Clear guidance is required if multiple observers are used • Time taken to collect data
Written records	• Researcher's influence is negligible, depending on the source of data • Views may be more freely expressed if outside a formal research setting (e.g. social media posts)	• Ethical aspects will need to be addressed if data was originally collected for another purpose • Important to ensure data use is public or approval has been obtained • Data may not be directly relevant to the research question

Source: Adapted from Tuckerman et al. (9).

Principles of data analysis

The intention of the data analysis in qualitative research is to synthesise the individual ideas and experiences into a model or theory of the experience of the group under study (Figure 5.1) (10). First, the interview is transcribed. The researcher carefully reads this to obtain a feel for the data. Small units of meaning (codes) are identified. These are then grouped based on their shared concepts to form 'primary categories'. Based on their perceived connections, primary groups are clustered into 'secondary groups'. From these, themes and interpretation are identified to build meaning from the data in the form of an explanation or model for the topic (e.g. a health behaviour) (Figure 5.2) (10).

In the study report, the research will describe the key findings and themes from the studies. These are often supported by the participants' quotes (Table 5.3) (10). A description of the analytical framework used should be described and referenced. Study findings are represented by a schematic representation to facilitate better conceptualisation. The overall analysis process is the same across all qualitative designs, though each has design-specific procedures.

Computer-assisted qualitative data analysis (CAQDAS)

CAQDAS are technologies which support data analysis in qualitative research (11). The main advantages are efficiency of data analysis and transparency. Learning to use the software can be a challenge, and there is heavy emphasis on coding. This can detract from the more reflective aspects of data analysis, which are intended to characterise methods such as descriptive phenomenology (11). Predicted helpful future uses include the generation of word clouds and other visualisations of qualitative data. This may facilitate bracketing and triangulation.

Bias in qualitative research

Reflexivity

It would be exceptional for a researcher to have no bias about the topic under study (Chapter 7). Reflexivity is a term used in qualitative research. It is a reflective approach in which the researcher accounts for their own bias, values, preferences and preconceptions about the topic both at the outset and during the study. Keeping a diary or journal is recognised as a means of reflexivity. Accounting for the reflexivity of the research team improves the credibility of the study. It should be included in the study report. Important sources of bias in qualitative research are shown in Table 5.4 (12).

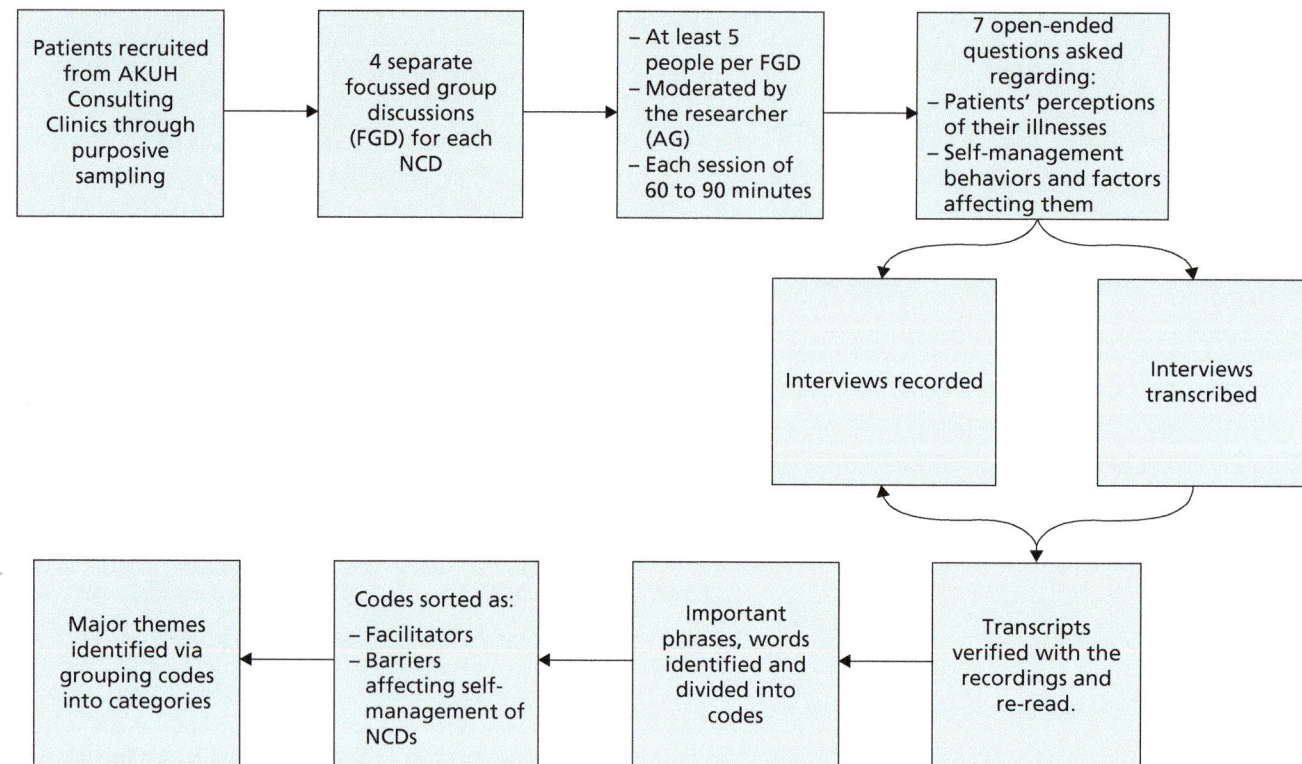

Figure 5.1 Qualitative study flow diagram illustrating the study processes. *Source:* Gowani et al. (10)/Springer Nature/CC BY 4.0.

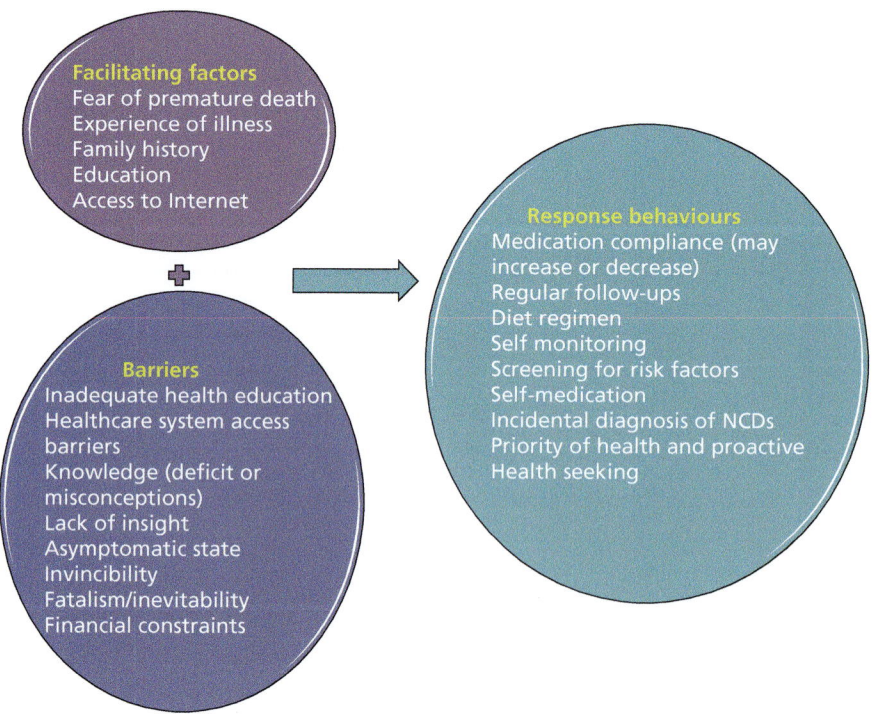

Figure 5.2 Conceptual framework of factors affecting non-communicable disease preventive behaviours. *Source:* Gowani et al. (10)/Springer Nature/CC BY 4.0.

Table 5.3 Qualitative themes and subcategories from the non-communicable disease (NCD) study.

Major themes	Categories	Subcategories	Excerpts from the patients' narratives
Factors affecting NCD preventive behaviours	*Positive factors/facilitators*	*Contributing actions*	*'I never miss my medications; they are most important to me'.*
	Fear of premature health Experience of illness	Medication compliance Follow-ups/checkups	*'My father had diabetes; I knew I will get it, so I had already controlled my intake of sugar'.*
	Familial inheritance of diseases Education level of the patient *Negative factors/barriers*	Diet regimen Self-monitoring *Contributing actions*	*'10 years ago, at the time of diagnosis, I did not know how much blood pressure was high, and how much was low. I learnt it over time, when I went through its fluctuating levels'.*
	Inadequate health education Healthcare system constraints Knowledge deficit	No regular screening Cost of the diagnostic tests Inability to interpret numeric values	
	Lack of insight about seriousness of disease	Self-medication	*'I stopped my medications after angioplasty for 2 years. . .had another heart attack and had a bypass then'.*
	No symptoms = no risk	Cholesterol screening not considered risk NCD diagnosed while seeking help for other medical conditions	
	Invincibility/lack of threat appreciation Unpredictability of disease Fatalism Finance	Sudden onset of acute events NCD are unpreventable Proactive help-seeking not a priority	*'I check BP and sugar regularly because alterations in it make me nonfunctional'.*
	Cost of fresh food, vegetables and unsaturated oil		

Source: Gowani et al. (10)/Springer Nature/CC BY 4.0.

Table 5.4 Sources of bias in qualitative research.

Recall bias Participants remember events or experiences inaccurately, leading to skewed data	*Confirmation bias* The tendency to seek information in a way that supports our existing beliefs while rejecting data which contradicts it	*Interview bias* Results from the researcher and the way they conduct the study. It can be the way they ask questions or react to answers but may also arise from the interviewer's personal characteristics
Procedural bias Participants are given insufficient time to respond to a question, interview or survey	*Selection bias* Distortion or skewing of research outcomes due to selection of a non-representative sample	*Sampling bias* Selection of participants for a study is not representative of the population in whom the results need to be applied
Acquiescence bias Tendency to agree with a statement when given a binary (e.g. Yes/No) response	*Design bias* The researcher's preferences dominate the design, survey questions and methodology rather than what is best for the research	*Observer bias* Attribution of participant behaviours to internal factors such as skills or personality, but researcher's own behaviour to external or situational factors
Question order bias The order of questions can affect the participant's replies	*Cultural bias* Research conducted in a limited cultural setting or where the researcher prioritises their own cultural values in interpreting the data emerging from a different culture	*Researcher bias* The researcher's preferences and choices have an undue influence on the design and conduct of the study

Halo effect
A tendency to view a participant's responses more positively because of the responses themselves or because of personal characteristics of the respondent.

Source: Adapted from Pannucci and Wilkins (12).

Reporting qualitative research studies

The Equator Network (https://www.equator-network.org) highlights two main guidelines for the reporting of qualitative research for publication: the Standards for Reporting Qualitative Research (SRQR) (13) and the Consolidated Criteria for Reporting Qualitative Research (COREQ) (14). Several reporting guidelines have been developed. One of the issues is any guideline's need to cover and reflect the varying methodologies of qualitative research. SRQR is based on a systematic review of existing guidelines, reporting standards and critical appraisal criteria. The final document aimed to provide an outline standard while allowing flexibility to incorporate the various approaches and methods (13). It enables authors to report to a standard while also facilitating critical appraisal, application and synthesis of findings.

Critical appraisal of qualitative research

There is some debate about whether and how to appraise qualitative research (15). One of the tenets of EBM is critical appraisal of research, especially where it relates to clinical decision-making and patient safety. Assessing the trustworthiness of qualitative research has been discussed earlier (5). Use of both approaches facilitates the answering of different but related questions. Appraisal of qualitative research needs to go beyond the checklist approach. Completion of a checklist does not fix methodological flaws. It also requires an evaluation of the methodology used, whether that methodology was appropriate and if it did indeed contribute to the theory or model developed and its suggested next steps in terms of application or as a basis for further, quantitative research. Particular attention needs to be given to participant selection; participants should be representative of the study population rather than 'good' participants. Data collection should encourage participants to elaborate in their own words until they have nothing left to say rather than respond in a limited way (i.e. yes/no or via closed questions). Finally, the researcher should demonstrate reflection on how their own perspectives and biases may have impacted the interpretation of the data.

Mixed methods

Given the complementary approach of qualitative and quantitative approaches to research, the potential of their application to a particular problem at the same time is self-evident. Use of both approaches facilitates the answering of different but related questions. A protocol can be developed to direct all dimensions of the research (16). Mixed-methods research can also be used as the basis for systematic reviews (17).

Generalisability of qualitative research

Generalisability is more likely to be a wider application of concepts rather than numerical. It may enable practitioners to adopt approaches in communicating information to patients (e.g. shared decision-making, communication of risk) (18).

References

1 Green, J. and Britten, N. (1998). Qualitative research and evidence based medicine. *BMJ* 316 (7139): 1230–1232.

2 Renjith, V., Yesodharan, R., Noronha, J.A. et al. (2021). Qualitative methods in health care research. *Int J Prev Med* 12: 20.

3 Munhall, P.L. (2012). *Nursing Research: A Qualitative Perspective* (ed. M.A. Sudbury). Jones and Barlett Leaning.

4 Omerovic, E., Petrie, M., Redfors, B. et al. (2024). Pragmatic randomized controlled trials: strengthening the concept through a robust international collaborative network: PRIME-9-Pragmatic Research and Innovation through Multinational Experimentation. *Trials* 25 (1): 80.

5 Williams, V., Boylan, A.M., and Nunan, D. (2020). Critical appraisal of qualitative research: necessity, partialities and the issue of bias. *BMJ Evid Based Med* 25 (1): 9–11.

6 Moorley, C. and Cathala, X. (2019). How to appraise qualitative research. *Evid Based Nurs* 22 (1): 10–13.

7 Strauss, A.C.J. (2014). *Basics of Qualitative Research Techniques and Procedures for Developing Grounded Theroy*. London: Sage.

8 Offredy, M.V.P. (2010). *Developing a Healthcare Research Proposal: An Interactive Student Guide*. Oxford: Wiley-Blackwell.

9 Tuckerman, J., Kaufman, J., and Danchin, M. (2020). How to use qualitative methods for health and health services research. *J Paediatr Child Health* 56 (5): 818–820.

10 Gowani, A., Ahmed, H.I., Khalid, W. et al. (2016). Facilitators and barriers to NCD prevention in Pakistanis-invincibility or inevitability: a qualitative research study. *BMC Res Notes* 9: 282.

11 Vignato, J., Inman, M., Patsais, M., and Conley, V. (2022). Computer-assisted qualitative data analysis software, phenomenology, and colaizzi's method. *West J Nurs Res* 44 (12): 1117–1123.

12 Pannucci, C.J. and Wilkins, E.G. (2010). Identifying and avoiding bias in research. *Plast Reconstr Surg* 126 (2): 619–625.

13 O'Brien, B.C., Harris, I.B., Beckman, T.J. et al. (2014). Standards for reporting qualitative research: a synthesis of recommendations. *Acad Med* 89 (9): 1245–1251.

14 Tong, A., Sainsbury, P., and Craig, J. (2007). Consolidated criteria for reporting qualitative research (COREQ): a 32-item checklist for interviews and focus groups. *Int J Qual Health Care* 19 (6): 349–357.

15 Majid, U. and Vanstone, M. (2018). Appraising qualitative research for evidence syntheses: a compendium of quality appraisal tools. *Qual Health Res* 28 (13): 2115–2131.

16 Cottrell, E., Darney, B.G., Marino, M. et al. (2019). Study protocol: a mixed-methods study of women's healthcare in the safety net after Affordable Care Act implementation - EVERYWOMAN. *Health Res Policy Syst* 17 (1): 58.

17 Jarva, E., Mikkonen, K., Tuomikoski, A.M. et al. (2021). Healthcare professionals' competence in stroke care pathways: a mixed-methods systematic review. *J Clin Nurs* 30 (9–10): 1206–1235.

18 Song, D., Zhou, J., Fan, T. et al. (2022). Decision aids for shared decision-making and appropriate anticoagulation therapy in patients with atrial fibrillation: a systematic review and meta-analysis. *Eur J Cardiovasc Nurs* 21 (2): 97–106.

19 Goff, S.L., Wallace, K., Putnam, N. et al. (2022). A qualitative study of health workers' experiences during early surges in the COVID-19 pandemic in the U.S.: implications for ongoing occupational health challenges. *Front Public Health* 10: 780711.

20 Butler, A., Hall, H., and Copnell, B. (2016). A guide to writing a qualitative systematic review protocol to enhance evidence-based practice in nursing and health care. *Worldviews Evid-Based Nurs* 13 (3): 241–249.

21 Hennink, M. and Kaiser, B.N. (2022). Sample sizes for saturation in qualitative research: a systematic review of empirical tests. *Soc Sci Med* 292: 114523.

CHAPTER 6

Statistical Concepts

John Frain

Division of Medical Sciences and Graduate Entry Medicine, University of Nottingham, UK

OVERVIEW

- Quantitative research generates numbers; statistics help us understand the meaning of these numbers.
- Statistics can be applied to describe data, generate a hypothesis or test a hypothesis.
- You should understand when and how statistical tests are applied.
- You should be able to interpret the reported results of statistical tests.
- Interpretation of statistics is important in assessing the quality of a study.
- There are common mistakes and misconceptions around statistics.

Introduction

When you practise evidence-based healthcare, you need to assess the quality of research. This enables you to decide when evidence is useful for your clinical decision-making. This chapter provides an overview of the overarching concepts in medical statistics. It will not be possible to cover all topics relevant to statistics for evidence-based healthcare. Interpreting and communicating risk are covered in Chapter 8. For a more detailed account of statistics for evidence-based healthcare, the reader is referred to the resources at the end of this book.

Oh no, not statistics!

Statistics is the method enabling collection, analysis, presentation and interpretation of numerical data. Confidence in interpreting statistics is related to previous good experience in the learning of mathematics. Previous poor learning experience facilitates ambivalence and apathy for statistics among students.

The origin of statistics dates from John Graunt's *Natural and Political Observations on the Bills of Mortality* in 1663. Graunt analysed weekly data on deaths in London to estimate the city's population, constructed the first-ever life table and identified there were more male than female births (ratio 107:100) (1).

What are statistics for?

Medical statistics concerns collecting, summarising and analysing data to draw conclusions about a population or group. This is based on the collection of data or variables about the population. Examples include age, sex, height, weight and blood pressure. Several types of statistics are used in research (Box 6.1).

Analysis, including the use of statistical tests, should be embedded in the planning, data collection, interpretation and reporting of research findings. Researchers must understand statistics to meticulously design epidemiological studies and clinical trials. Clinicians need knowledge of statistics to properly interpret the results of research for application in practice.

Types of data

Individual characteristics such as age, height, weight, gender identity and hair colour are variables. Data is the value placed on each one. You need to know what form your data takes to analyse it. Data is either:
- Numerical (quantitative) – age, height and weight
- Categorical (qualitative) – gender identity and hair colour

Choice of statistical test depends on whether data are categorical or numerical. Identifying the type of data you have guides how it is analysed. Data can be visualised (e.g. in a graph).

Identifying data types

Numerical (quantitative) data

Numerical data is data recorded as numbers. These variables can be added, subtracted, multiplied or divided. Numerical biological data include age, blood pressure, body mass index (BMI), pulse and respiratory rate. Numerical data can be categorised further into *continuous* or *discrete* types.

Continuous – there is no limitation on the values that the variables can take – they can take on any value within a given range, e.g. weight (73 or 80.4 kg) or height (1.67 m or 180 cm).

Discrete – the variable can only take on certain whole numerical values, e.g. the number of children in a family – you can only have 0, 1, 2, 3, 4, 5, etc., or the number of wheels on a car (i.e. 4).

ABC of Evidence-Based Healthcare, First Edition. Edited by John Frain.

In practical terms, we do not often distinguish between the two. For example, the average British family has 2.7 children. In this calculation, discrete numerical data have been analysed as if they were continuous.

Categorical data

Categorical (qualitative) data – categories (not numbers)
1 Binary = two categories, e.g. Yes/No, Dead/Alive and Disease/No Disease
  a You can assign the values to these categories and do some numerical analysis (e.g. Yes = 1 and No = 2)
2 Nominal = more than two categories that have no order
  a Blood groups (A, B, AB and O)
  b Marital status (single, married and divorced)
3 Ordinal = more than two categories that have a specific order
  a Example: Disease staging systems
    i 0 = carcinoma in situ
    ii 1 = localised cancer
    iii 2 = advanced local cancer
    iv 3 = advanced local cancer
    v 4 = metastatic cancer

Descriptive and inferential statistics

As well as individual subjects, the researcher is interested in how variables across groups of individuals (populations or samples) change and what this might mean for health. Simple examples are weight and height. Variables of clinical interest might be how blood pressure varies with age, as this is important for diagnosis and treatment in at-risk groups. Descriptive statistics describe the relationship between variables in a sample or population. Put simply, they answer the basic questions about a study population: who, what, why, when and where? (2)

Descriptive statistics also assess the central tendency of data to cluster around a central value within the range of possible values. For example, while height is a continuous variable in adults, there is a lower and an upper limit, with most people's height being 'in the middle' or average for the population (174.4 cm for males and 162.4 cm for females in the United Kingdom in 2021) (3). Central tendency is the statistical measure that identifies a single value that is most typical or representative of an entire distribution. Measures of central tendency are mean, median and mode (Box 6.2).

The most used measure of central tendency is the mean. The advantage of the mean is that it uses every value in the data in its calculation. Repeated samples drawn from the same population tend to have similar means. The mean is the best measure of central tendency, which best resists the fluctuation between samples. A single value representing a complete data set (e.g. a group of patients) is useful as it facilitates comparison between groups.

Comparison of groups, for example, the intervention and control groups of a randomised controlled trial (RCT), is a key concept in medical statistics. Comparison between groups facilitates inferential (exploratory and confirmatory) statistics where the evidence for modelling of disease and treatment data is explored and confirmed. Inferential statistics use data from a random sample from a population which is intended to be representative of the entire population (Chapter 4). The tests used describe and allow inferences about the variable (e.g. blood pressure) in the entire population. Inferential statistics are essential in research where it is not possible to include every member of the population.

A disadvantage of the mean is its sensitivity to extreme values (outliers) in a data set, especially when the sample is small. It is useful where data are normally distributed. Where the data are skewed, the mean is not an appropriate measure of central tendency. The mean cannot be calculated for nominal or non-nominal ordinal data. Even where it can be calculated, it does not necessarily provide a meaningful value (e.g. stage of cancer).

Measures of spread of data

Data variability or dispersion (spread) is a measure of how much recorded observations in a data set differ from one another. Range, standard deviation and interquartile range (IR) are all measures of how the data is spread around its central point (Box 6.3). The standard deviation is usually reported for the mean and IR for a median value.

Box 6.3 **Measures of data variability or dispersion**

Range – the difference between the largest and the smallest value.
Advantages – it is easily determined.
Disadvantages – it only uses two observations, and it is distorted by outliers and tends to increase with increasing sample size.
Variance – reports how much *each observation* deviates from the mean. The larger the deviation from the mean, the greater the variability in the observations.
Advantage – it can be calculated easily for data collected from the entire population (divide by 'n') or a sample of the population (divide by '$n-1$').
Disadvantage – the final value is a square of the raw data (standard deviation corrects this).

Standard deviation
Standard deviation is the average of the *deviations* from the mean (as calculated by variance).

It is the most reported measure of variability. In calculations, it is noted as σ and is the *square root* of the variance.

Advantages – uses every observation and algebraically defined
Disadvantages – sensitive to outliers and inappropriate for skewed data

Percentiles and interquartile range
Observations are ranked, with the middle line representing the median (50th percentile).

Minimum and maximum values are represented. The distance from the 25th to 75th percentile is reported as the interquartile range.

Advantage – suitable for reporting skewed data
Disadvantage – gives quite basic measures of spread

Reporting central tendency

Central tendency should always be reported. Appropriate reporting depends on the spread of the data. With symmetrical distribution of data (normal distribution), the mean, median and mode should all be identical. In this case, the mean should be reported as it is a more accurate measure. With a skewed distribution of data, the mean and median will be different. Now, the median is more appropriate as it is less affected by the skew than is the mean.

Visualising data

Visualising data on a graph is especially useful for getting a 'feel' for the data. A graph is useful for spotting outliers (unusual results). It provides a clear summary of the data, describes how the data are distributed and helps to identify trends. The normal distribution is one of the most important distributions in statistics (Figure 6.1). It is bell-shaped, symmetrical about the mean (mean = median) and defined by the mean and standard deviation. If data is 'perfectly,' normally distributed, the probability of a variable falling within:

$\pm$1 standard deviation of the mean is ~68%
$\pm$1.96 standard deviations of the mean is ~95%
$\pm$2.58 standard deviations of the mean is ~99%

However, data are not commonly, normally distributed in medicine. Deviations from normality are described in relation to the skew of the data and the kurtosis (shape) of the curve. Data can be positively (skew to the right) or negatively (skew to the left) skewed. The skew direction describes the position of the 'tail' of the curve and *not* the position of the peak of the curve. In non-normal data distributions, mean, median and mode have different values, and the mean is taken as the value of interest for further analysis (Figure 6.2) (2). There are several types of graphs. The central tendency and dispersion of data applies in all of them (Figure 6.3).

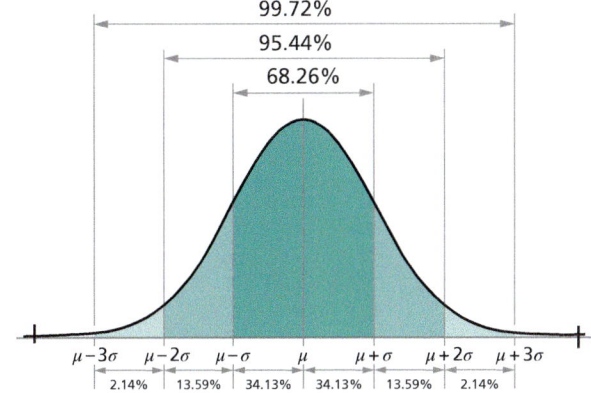

Figure 6.1 The normal distribution showing symmetrical data dispersion (spread) on either side of the mean using the standard deviation. In a normal (Gaussian) distribution, mean, median and mode all have the same value. (where μ = mean and σ = standard deviation). *Source:* Shutterstock standard licence.

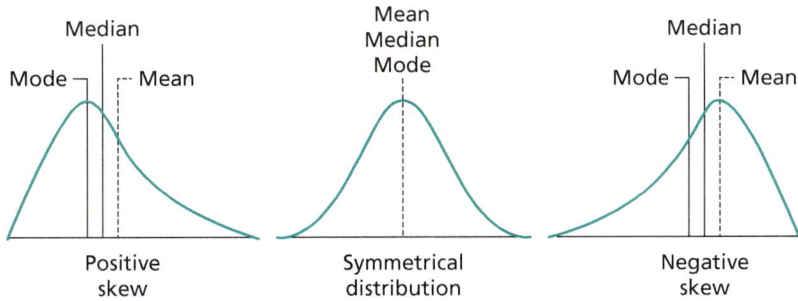

Figure 6.2 Non-normal data distribution. *Source:* Adapted from Alatefi et al. (4).

(a)

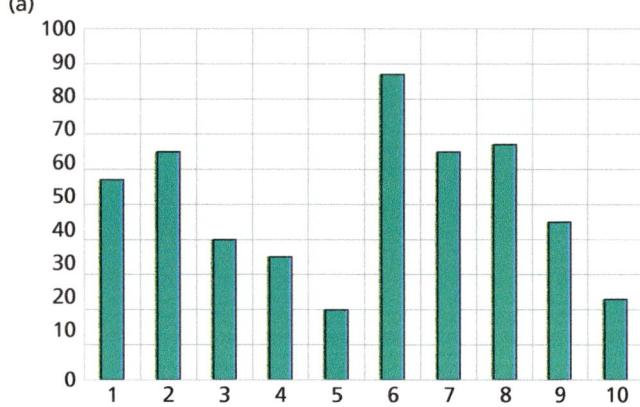

(b)

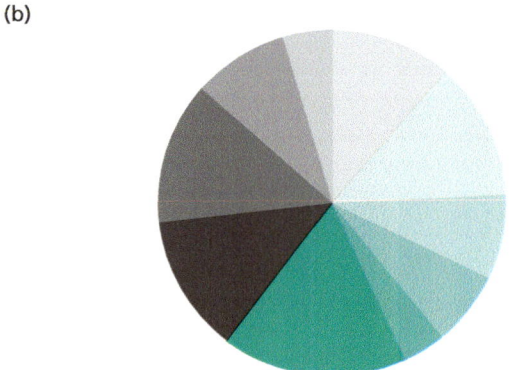

(c)

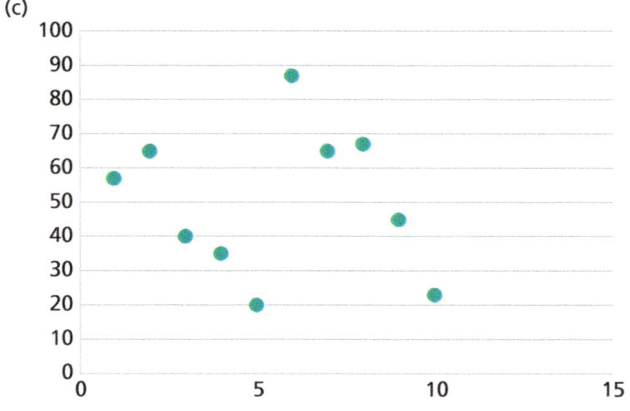

(d)

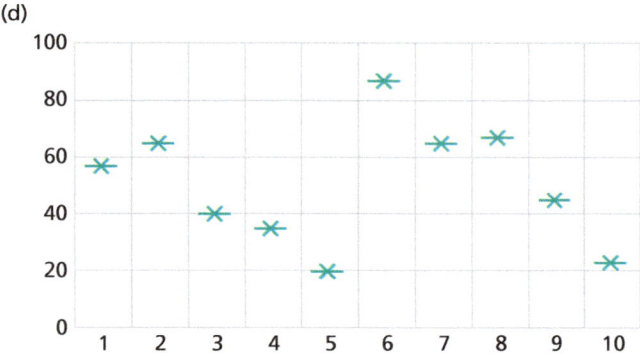

Figure 6.3 Examples of charts used to visualise data. These charts all contain the same data. (a) Bar chart, (b) Pie chart, (c) Scatter, (d) Box and whisker.

Transforming data

Why would you want to transform data? Transformation takes data which are not normally distributed and converts the data into normally distributed data. A more rigorous analysis can be performed if data are normally distributed. The mathematical transformation used is applied to each piece of raw data. The most used technique is the log transformation. Other transformation techniques include square root transformation, reciprocal transformation, square transformation and logistic transformation.

Sample point estimate (2)

Using random sampling, the estimated value of a parameter for a group at a point in time can be estimated. The sample is selected from within a larger population of interest. Calculation of the mean provides a value of a variable within a group, which can be used to estimate the corresponding population value. A repeated series of random samples of data from the same underlying population would be expected to produce a different yet equally valid point estimate of the corresponding population estimate. This can be calculated for every group. It allows comparison of groups. For example, two groups could be compared where one had received a medical intervention and one had not.

Data accuracy and quality

Accuracy is how closely a measurement detects the 'true' value. Precision is the consistency and repeatability of a measurement, regardless of the accuracy of measurement.

Errors, bias and prejudice

No data are absolutely precise and accurate. Box 6.4 shows some common statistical causes of error in research. Other causes include competing interests, commercial interests and those who set out to 'prove' or 'disprove' something.

Standard error

A large standard error indicates that the estimate generated by the study is *imprecise*. Standard error is reduced if the sample size is increased, and there is less data variability. A random sample should be used whenever possible to reduce the chance of bias. If this is not practical, a convenience sample can be taken. For example, when

Box 6.4 **Causes of measurement error**

- Measurement/equipment error
- Errors intrinsic to the procedure
- Operator errors – training, consistency of approach and record keeping
- Non-random sampling
- Interference by the process of investigation
- Investigator bias – conscious or unconscious

studying patients with a particular clinical condition, you may choose to examine patients in a particular hospital. However, this can increase the standard error – a balance needs to be struck between using an appropriate sample and reducing potential standard error.

Standard error of the mean

Since comparison of groups relies on the mean, the standard error of the mean (SEM) is important. If we take multiple samples from the UK population (weight of elderly men in the UK cities of Derby, Nottingham, Birmingham, etc.), each has a slightly different sample mean. These sample means will be distributed about the actual UK population mean. The SEM is the standard deviation (variability) of these sample means. It tells us how well our single city samples represent the UK population. If the SEM is large, then our sample is probably not representative of the overall population.

Standard deviation (SD) or standard error of the mean (SEM) – which should I use?

a SD describes variability in the data values – use this to show variability in the data (e.g. lab-based research articles).
b SEM describes precision of the sample mean – use when interested in the mean of a set of data values (e.g. clinical study-based research articles).

Confidence intervals

How sure are you of your results? This is the fundamental question when analysing data, and confidence intervals are the way to answer it.

The confidence interval (CI) of a mean tells you how precisely you have determined the mean, i.e. how close is your sample mean to the true population mean? Generation of the CI values is achieved by combining sample size and variability (standard deviation) for the population mean. As its name suggests, the CI is a range of values.

Confidence intervals of a mean

Sampling error occurs during sample selection. However, we can estimate a margin of error to reflect this uncertainty. CIs define boundaries within which we can confidently expect the population to fall. To interpret CIs, you must assume the values are normally distributed.

In a normally distributed sample set, the CI provides us with a range of values in which we are 95% confident that the true population mean lies (and do not include the population in the other 5%). Ninety-five percent of the distribution of sample means lies within ± 1.96 standard deviations of the population mean.

Why do we use 95%?

You can use any percentage CI, but 95% is standard. If you use other percentage CI: 99% CI will be wider, 90% CI will be narrower and 50% CI will be very narrow. If you want more confidence that an interval contains the true parameter, then the intervals will be wider. If you want to be 100% sure that an interval contains the true population, it must contain every value and so be infinitely wide. If you are willing to be only 50% sure that an interval contains the true value, then it can be much narrower – but this is not good practice, and you would question this in a research paper.

Hypothesis testing

Hypotheses are used in experimental design studies such as RCTs. Hypothesis testing is used to investigate relationships between variables or, more commonly in healthcare, to test for differences between groups.

For example, you are testing the efficacy of a new drug for treatment of depression and have a study with three groups of participants:

a Traditional treatment
b Control (no treatment)
c Novel treatment

Having collected your data from all participants, you would use a statistical measure/test to look to see if there are any significant differences between the groups. Most statistical tests generate some sort of test statistic and a *P* value.

The null hypothesis

To test a hypothesis, firstly you must generate your *null* hypothesis. A null hypothesis (H_0) assumes *no effect* – there is no difference between the means of the groups (so all differences are due to random sampling). For example, if comparing rates of smoking between men and women in the population, the null hypothesis would be:

H_0 – smoking rates are the same in men and women in the population

The alternative hypothesis (H_1) assumes there is an effect so:

H_1 – smoking rates are different in men and women in the population

Statistical testing is performed on the null hypothesis, and it tells us whether to accept or reject the null hypothesis. Therefore, the alternative hypothesis will hold only if the null hypothesis is rejected.

Errors in hypothesis testing

Errors in hypothesis testing occur due to incorrect use and interpretation of statistical tests. It is important to understand when and why each test should be used to ensure you are using the correct one, but also that the correct analysis was carried out in the literature you are using.

Type 1 error

A false positive – rejecting the null hypothesis incorrectly, i.e. concluding there is a difference where none exists.

Type 2 error

A false negative – failure to reject the null hypothesis, i.e. failure to detect a difference where one exists.

Type 1 errors are more severe than type 2 errors. When analysing data, you do not know the population mean, so you cannot know whether a particular CI contains the true population mean or not. All you know is that there is a 95% chance that the CI includes the population mean and a 5% chance that it does not. With a large sample, you know the mean with much more precision than with a small sample; therefore, the CI is quite narrow.

What is a *P* value?

It is the probability of observing the differences in your sample simply by chance. Almost every statistical test generates a *P* value (or several).

$P < 0.05$ means <5% probability of the results arising by chance
$P < 0.01$ means <1% probability of the results arising by chance
$P < 0.001$ means <0.1% probability of the results arising by chance

A sufficiently small *P* value allows the null hypothesis to be rejected. In the medical sciences, we adopt a threshold of $p < 0.05$, that is, you would expect on 5% of occasions that you would see an effect as extreme as the one that you observed if the null hypothesis were true. For example, you compared 2 means and obtained a *P* value of 0.02 means: There is a 2% chance of observing a difference as large as you observed even if both population groups are identical/the null hypothesis is true. This allows you to reject the null hypothesis and state that the results are statistically significant. In this context, the term 'significant' should only be related to statistical or clinical significance.

Choosing statistical tests

Statistical tests are used in healthcare research to compare means between groups or to compare percentages or proportions between groups. Choice of test will be different in each type of comparison. Tests may be either parametric or non-parametric. For parametric statistics, the study outcome data follow a normal distribution, and

the variances in each of the groups are equal. In non-parametric test, outcome data do not follow a normal distribution.

The groups compared may be independent or dependent. For independent groups, participants in one group do not provide information about subjects in another group. In dependent groups, data may be collected at two different points in time, for example, pre- and post-treatment. An alternative scenario is, for example, in case-control studies where subjects in one group have been matched to individuals in another group (e.g. age and medical condition). Figures 6.4 and 6.5 outline how to choose a test to compare groups.

Correlation and regression

Inferential statistics also explore the relationship between variables (Table 6.1). Correlation analysis is used to explore the strength of association between variables where neither is assumed to predict the occurrence of the other. For normally distributed data, the parametric test is Pearson correlation coefficient (*r*), where the result ranges from −1 to +1. The non-parametric test is Spearman correlation coefficient. Again, results range from −1 to +1 with 0 indicating no correlation.

Regression analysis can be used only when one variable is thought to change the other. This may be a linear relationship where an explanatory variable (*x*) influences a dependent variable (*y*). Multiple regression analysis permits investigation of several explanatory variables on a dependent variable. Logistic regression is like linear regression except the dependent variable has a binary outcome. This is used to explore whether a risk factor for a disease (e.g. hyperlipidaemia) predicts the development of a disease or not (e.g. ischaemic heart disease).

Population and sampling

The population is the entire group in whom we are interested. It is usually impossible to study the entire population (cost, time, practicality, etc.). Therefore, we collect data from a sample of the

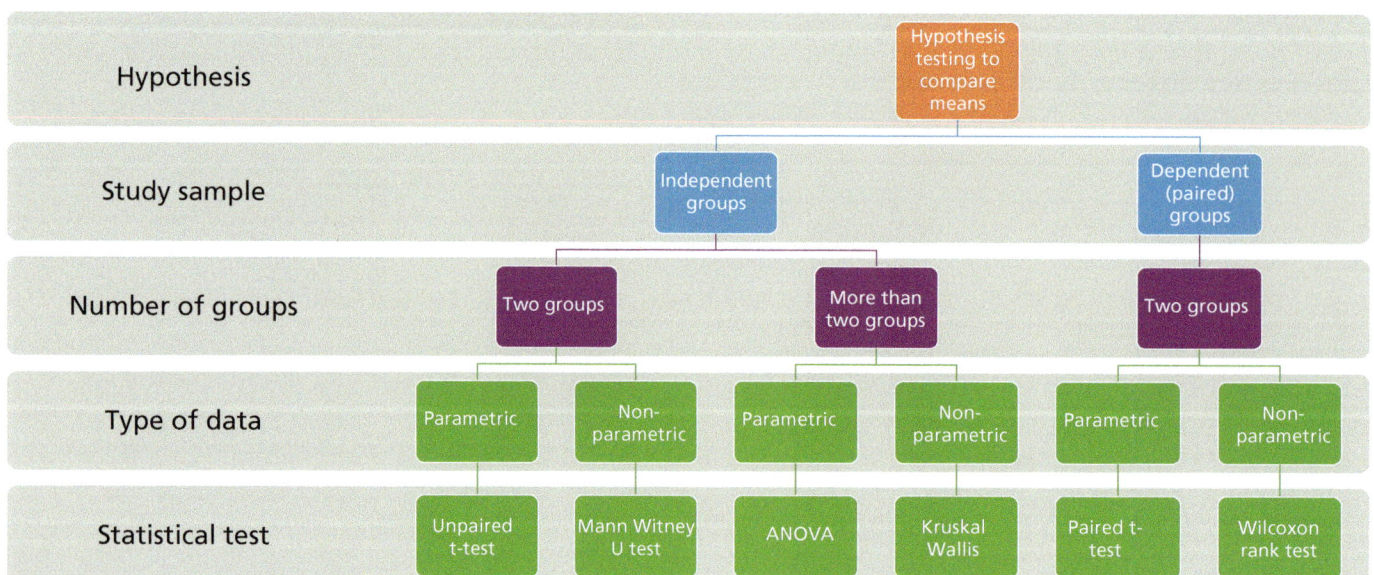

Figure 6.4 Choice of test for comparing the means of two groups. *Source:* Adapted from Biddle et al. (2023).

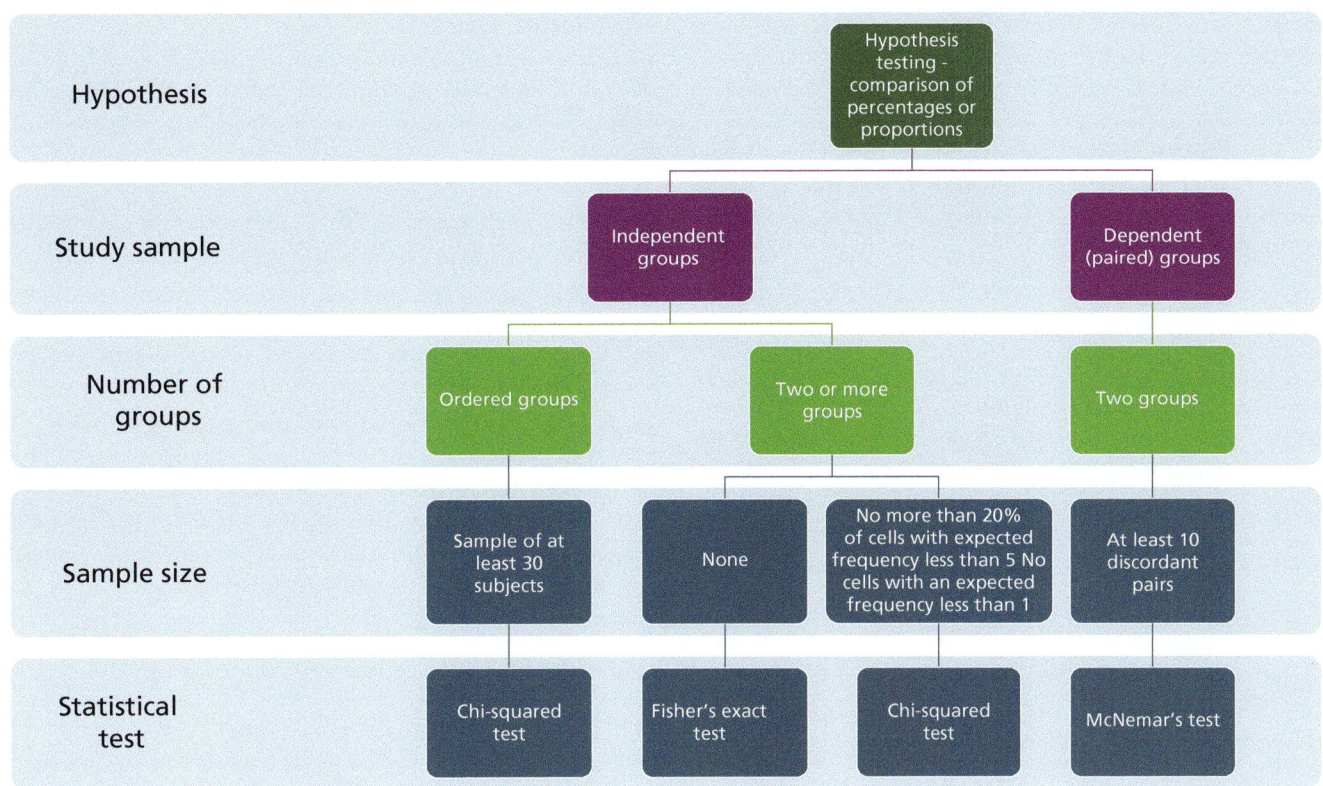

Figure 6.5 Choice of test for comparison of proportions or percentages between two groups. *Source:* Adapted from Biddle et al. (2023).

Table 6.1 Examples of studies of correlation and regression (5–8).

Correlation
Abdelbasset, W.K., Alsubaie, S.F., Tantawy, S.A. et al. (2019). A cross-sectional study on the correlation between physical activity levels and health-related quality of life in community-dwelling middle-aged and older adults. *Medicine (Baltimore)* 98 (11): e14895. https://doi.org/10.1097/MD.0000000000014895. PMID: 30882705; PMCID: PMC6426542.

High and moderate levels of physical activity have a great positive relationship with the health-related quality of life (HRQoL) in community-dwelling middle-aged and older adults in Egypt. Recommendations should be dedicated to supporting the active lifestyle among the different populations, particularly middle-aged and older adults.

Linear regression
Edelman, E.R., van Kuijk, S.M.J., Hamaekers, A.E.W. et al. (2017). Improving the Prediction Of Total Surgical Procedure Time Using Linear Regression Modeling. *Front Med (Lausanne)* 4: 85. https://doi.org/10.3389/fmed.2017.00085. PMID: 28674693; PMCID: PMC5475434.

Total procedure time (TPT) was most accurately predicted using a linear regression model based on the independent variables estimated surgeon-controlled time (eSCT), type of operation, American Society of Anaesthesiologists (ASA) classification and type of anaesthesia. This model performed significantly better than the fixed ratio model and the method of predicting anaesthesia-controlled time (ACT) separately.

Multiple regression
Trunfio, T.A., Scala, A., Giglio, C. et al. (2022). Multiple regression model to analyze the total LOS for patients undergoing laparoscopic appendectomy. *BMC Med Inform Decis Mak* 22 (1): 141. https://doi.org/10.1186/s12911-022-01884-9. PMID: 35610697; PMCID: PMC9131683.

This work designed an effective and automated strategy for improving the prediction of length of stay (LOS) that can be useful for enhancing the preoperative pathways. In this way it is possible to characterise the demand and to be able to estimate a priori the occupation of the beds and other related hospital resources.

Logistical regression
Bertoncelli, C.M., Altamura, P., Vieira, E.R. et al. (2020). PredictMed: a logistic regression-based model to predict health conditions in cerebral palsy. *Health Informatics J* 26 (3): 2105–2118. https://doi.org/10.1177/1460458219898568. Epub 2020 Jan 20. PMID: 31957544.

Our model represents a novelty in the field of some cerebral palsy-related health outcomes treatment, and it should significantly help doctors' decision-making process regarding patient prognosis.

population and use this to draw conclusions about the wider population. This information may not fully reflect the population, which introduces sampling error, reported as the standard error. The sample size needs to be carefully determined if you are using it to make inferences about your population. Power analysis is used to calculate the minimum sample size needed to detect an effect being investigated (e.g. effect of a new medication to treat depression).

The power of a study is the likelihood it will detect a clinically significant difference between groups, if one exists. It is usually set at 80–90%. Increasing sample size increases the study's power. The larger the effect size, the easier it will be to detect a difference between the groups. Increased variability of outcome data decreases statistical power. Larger levels of significance level increase the power of a study but also the chance of a Type 2 error.

Diagnostic tests

Although diagnosis is one of the key outcomes in healthcare, there is no perfect test.

Sensitivity and specificity are commonly used to assess test utility. This is most easily calculated in the 2×2 table which outlines the frequency of those having the disease of interest (Table 6.2).

The perfect test would be 100% sensitive (it would be positive in all patients with the disease) and 100% specific (it would be positive only in patients with the disease). However, in real life some patients will have positive test results but not have the disease (false positives), while others will have negative results but in fact have the disease (false negatives). The threshold (cut-off point) for a test is set using a level where the resulting sensitivity and specificity of the test result reflect the nature of the target disease. In clinical practice, more sensitive tests are less specific, while more specific tests are less sensitive. For serious diseases which are treatable, greater sensitivity enables more patients to be diagnosed, even though some patients will have initially positive results and be further investigated unnecessarily.

Individual test sensitivity and specificity are not 'usable' by the bedside. Further calculations which can facilitate a diagnosis are predictive values, likelihood ratios (LRs) and ROC (receiver operating characteristic) curves.

Table 6.2 Calculation of sensitivity and specificity using a 2×2 table.

Test result	Disease	No disease
Positive	a	b
Negative	c	d

Sensitivity is the proportion of subjects who do not have the condition and have a negative test result. It is calculated from:

Sensitivity = $d/b + d$

Specificity is the proportion of subjects who do have the disease and who also have a positive test result. Calculation is from:

Specificity = $a/a + c$

Predictive values

These are dependent on the prevalence of the disease in the population being tested. For common conditions, the PPV (positive predictive value) is higher than in populations where the disease is rare.

$$\text{Positive predictive value}\left(\text{PPV}\right) = \text{the proportion of individuals with a positive test result who } do \text{ have the disease} = a/\left(a+b\right)$$

$$\text{Negative predictive value}\left(\text{NPV}\right) = \text{proportion of individuals with a negative test result who } do \, not \text{ have the disease} = c/\left(c+d\right)$$

Likelihood ratios and pre- and post-test odds

Pre- and post-test probability of a patient having the target disease is the odds before and after a diagnostic test is performed. It is uncommon to know the exact pre-test probability of a patient having a condition before the diagnostic test is performed. Usually, the pre-test probability of the individual patient is assumed to be the same as the general population or:

$$\text{Pre-test probability} = \text{prevalence}\left(1 - \text{prevalence}\right)$$

The post-test odds (probability) following a positive test depend on both the pre-test odds and LR of the test, where:

$$\text{Post-test odds} = \text{pre-test odds} \times \text{LR}$$

An LR provides a measure of the performance of a test. Since the value of an LR does not depend on the prevalence of the target condition, it has greater utility 'by the bedside' when assessing patients. It is calculated by:

$$\text{LR} = \text{sensitivity}/\left(1 - \text{specificity}\right)$$

When the LR is greater than 1, the test is more likely to give a positive result if the patient has the disease than if they did not. The greater the LR, the greater the discriminatory power of the test (Figures 6.6 and 6.7). In Figure 6.6, the percentages displayed indicate the increase in probability of the condition being diagnosed given the value of the LR.

Receiving operating characteristic (ROC) curves

A ROC curve is used to determine the most appropriate cut-off value (threshold) for a diagnostic test (i.e. the value at which the test is categorised as positive). It is a plot of sensitivity (y) versus ($1 - \text{specificity}$) on the x-axis (Figure 6.8). The greater the discrimination of the test, the closer the curve lies to the upper left-hand corner of the graph. The area under the curve (AUC) gives a combined measure of the sensitivity and specificity of the test and thus its validity. An AUC of 1 means the test discriminates perfectly between individuals with the disease and those without the disease. An AUC of 0.5 (straight line) indicates the result of the test is due to chance. Validated tests have AUC values between 0.5 and 1.0. This method enables comparison of the accuracy of diagnostic tests.

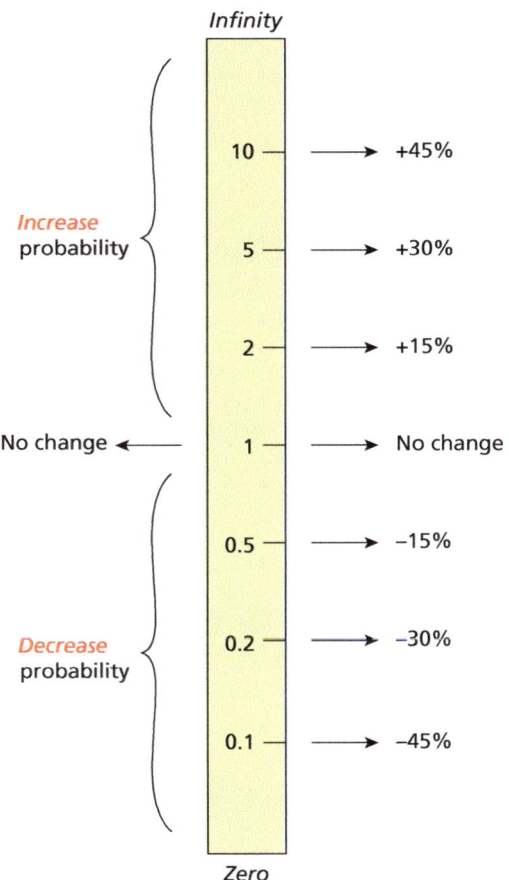

Infinity

Increase probability

No change ← → No change

Decrease probability

Zero

10 → +45%

5 → +30%

2 → +15%

1

0.5 → −15%

0.2 → −30%

0.1 → −45%

Figure 6.6 Likelihood ratios: diagnostic weights. Clinicians should classify LRs into three groups: those with values greater than 1.0 increase probability, those with values less than 1.0 decrease probability, and those with values near 1.0 change probability very little or not at all. *Source:* ABC of Clinical Reasoning, 2023/John Wiley & Sons.

(1) *Detecting pneumonia:* In patient with acute respiratory complaints, 'percussion dullness' is found in 18% of patients with pneumonia and in 6% of patients with another cause of respiratory distress. Therefore,

$$LR \binom{\text{for percussion dullness}}{\text{in detecting pneumonia}} = \frac{18}{6} = 3.0$$

(2) *Detecting coronary artery disease:* In patients with chronic chest pain, 'dysphagia' is reported in 4% of patients found to have coronary disease and in 20% of patients with another cause of chest pain. Therefore,

$$LR \left(\begin{array}{c} \text{for dysphagia} \\ \text{in detecting coronary} \\ \text{artery disease} \end{array} \right) = \frac{4}{20} = 0.2$$

Figure 6.7 Likelihood ratios: examples. From McGee, S. Likelihood ratios, definition and examples. In: Evidence-based physical diagnosis 5th Ed. Elsevier, 2021. *Source:* ABC of Clinical Reasoning, 2023/John Wiley & Sons.

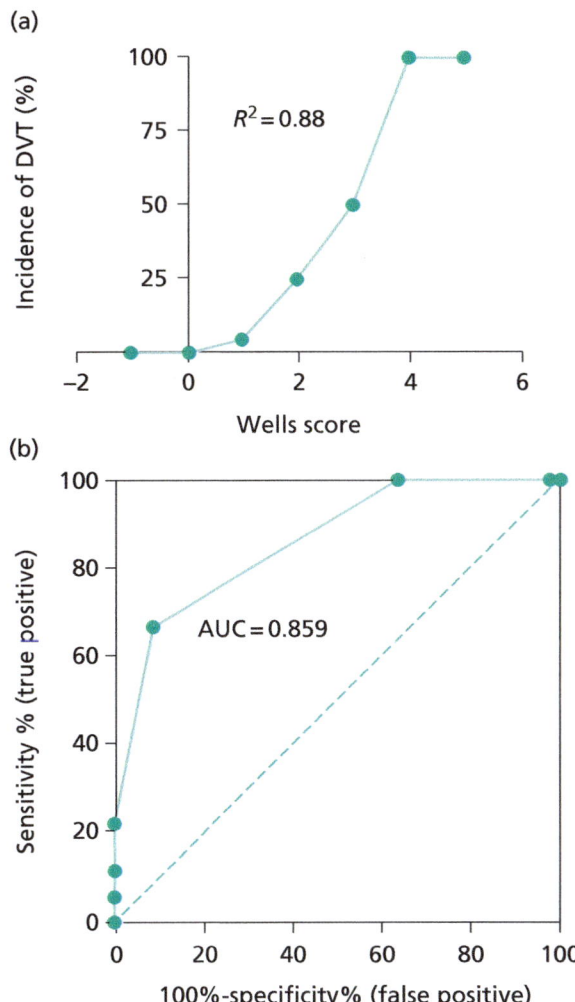

(a)

$R^2 = 0.88$

(b)

AUC = 0.859

Figure 6.8 ROC demonstrating diagnostic accuracy of Well score in the diagnosis of deep venous thrombosis (DVT) correlation between Wells score and incidence of DVT with coefficient of determination ($R^2 = 0.88$, $p = 0.0016$) demonstrating a strong linear correlation. (a) Receiver operating characteristic (ROC) curve demonstrating the performance of Wells score in predicting likelihood of DVT. (b) Area under the ROC curve (AUROCC) value shows that high Wells scoring system is efficient in identifying the patients at risk for developing DVT based on their estimated probability after trauma. *Source:* Modi et al. (9)/Springer Nature/CC BY 4.0.

References

1 Aggarwal, R. (2018). Statistical literacy for healthcare professionals: why is it important? *Ann Card Anaesth* 21 (4): 349–350.

2 Vetter, T.R. (2017). Descriptive statistics: reporting the answers to the 5 basic questions of who, what, why, when, where, and a sixth, so what? *Anesth Analg* 125 (5): 1797–1802.

3 Stewart, C. (2024). Height of individuals in England 19989-2021, by gender. https://www.statista.com/statistics/332542/height-of-individuals-by-gender-in-england-uk/#:~:text=According%20to%20the%20survey%2C%20the,up%20from%20161%20in%201998.

4 Alatefi, M., Ahmad, S., and Alkahtani, M. (2019). Performance evaluation using multivariate non-normal process capability. *Processes* 7 (11): 833. https://doi.org/10.3390/pr7110833.

5 Abdelbasset, W.K., Alsubaie, S.F., Tantawy, S.A. et al. (2019). A cross-sectional study on the correlation between physical activity levels and health-related quality of life in community-dwelling middle-aged and older adults. *Medicine (Baltimore)* 98 (11): e14895.

6 Edelman, E.R., van Kuijk, S.M.J., Hamaekers, A.E.W. et al. (2017). Improving the prediction of total surgical procedure time using linear regression modeling. *Front Med (Lausanne)* 4: 85.

7 Trunfio, T.A., Scala, A., Giglio, C. et al. (2022). Multiple regression model to analyze the total LOS for patients undergoing laparoscopic appendectomy. *BMC Med Inform Decis Mak* 22 (1): 141.

8 Bertoncelli, C.M., Altamura, P., Vieira, E.R. et al. (2020). PredictMed: a logistic regression-based model to predict health conditions in cerebral palsy. *Health Informatics J* 26 (3): 2105–2118.

9 Modi, S., Deisler, R., Gozel, K. et al. (2016). Wells criteria for DVT is a reliable clinical tool to assess the risk of deep venous thrombosis in trauma patients. *World J Emerg Surg* 8 (11): 24. https://doi.org/10.1186/s13017-016-0078-1. PMID: 27279896; PMCID: PMC4898382.

Further reading

Biddle, K., Blundell, A., and Sofat, N. (2023). *Understanding Clinical Research: An Introduction*. Banbury: Scion Publishing Ltd.

Kirkwood, B.R. and Sterne, J.A.C. (2025). *Essential Medical Statistics*, 3e. Oxford: Wiley-Blackwell.

Salkind, N.J. and Frey, B.B. (2019). *Statistics for People Who (Think they) Hate Statistics*, 7e. Thousand Oaks, CA: Sage.

CHAPTER 7

Critical Appraisal

John Frain

Division of Medical Sciences and Graduate Entry Medicine, University of Nottingham, Nottingham, UK

OVERVIEW

- Critical appraisal skills are crucial for every clinician and health policymaker.
- This chapter is about critical appraisal, evaluation, synthesis and recommendation for practice.
- A structured approach to critical appraisal is most effective.
- It includes assessing the compliance with reporting standards of individual studies.
- Tools are available to facilitate critical appraisal.

What is critical appraisal?

Critical appraisal is carefully and systematically examining research evidence to judge its trustworthiness, value and relevance in a particular context (1). It allows clinicians to use research evidence reliably and efficiently. Research studies do not give the same results – even in the same population using a similar or identical design. Results may even conflict with one another. No matter how accurate, research must be transferable/translatable into practice. In part, this is due to the research setting being different from the clinical environment. Clinical decision-making is often based on the findings of research studies. It is essential that clinicians assess the reliability of research. Structured critical appraisal enables a clinician to decide which research findings apply to their patient or population in their setting. It enables discrimination between good- and poor-quality research. The first step is to understand the type of study to search for in relation to your clinical query (Table 7.1) (1).

Ensuring the study identified has used a design suitable for the research question is crucial (Chapter 2). For example, where objective evidence of the safety of a new surgical procedure is required, the appropriate study is a randomised controlled trial (RCT). The more subjective qualitative study exploring the patient experience of having a new surgical procedure may generate hypotheses about the acceptability to patients of the new technique, but it will not establish whether the new procedure is safe for patients.

Similarly, a cross-sectional survey is helpful for determining the frequency of a condition (e.g. cancer) at a particular point in time, but it tells us nothing about the prognosis for patients living with cancer. In fact, the survey would be biased on the question of the prognosis for cancer, as it would include only patients with cancer who were alive and none of those who had already died (1). The appropriate study for this prognosis question is a cohort study, specifically an inception cohort where a newly diagnosed patient is entered into the study and followed up over time to find what happens to them.

Once suitable information has been retrieved, there are three key initial steps to take with each study identified:

- Is the research trustworthy? (validity)
- What is the research telling us? (results and conclusions)
- How useful is the research in the context of your work? (relevance)

Validity

The validity of a research study results has two aspects – internal validity and external validity.

Internal validity is how accurately the study achieves its aims and measures the outcome it sets out to measure. Was the method chosen by the investigators robust enough to answer the study question? This may not be immediately apparent on initial perusal of the study or reading the abstract but should be clear by the time the article has been critically appraised.

External validity is the extent to which the results are generalisable to the population more generally. In other words, would repeating a study in a population in a non-research setting achieve the same results? To improve external validity, researchers will try to design clinical trials mirroring real clinical environments, including the range of patients recruited, and by studying interventions which are realistic in practice (2).

It is not a given that a study with internal validity will have external validity. The opposite may sometimes be true. An example of the relationship between the two is an RCT testing the effect of prone versus supine positioning ventilation on mortality in patients

---

Table 7.1 Initial appraisal of different study designs.

Clinical questions	Clinical relevance and suggested best method of investigation
Aetiology/question	What caused the disorder, and how is this related to the development of illness?
	Example – case-control study – cohort study
Therapy	Which treatments do more good than harm compared with an alternative treatment?
	Example – randomised controlled trial, systematic review and meta-analysis
Prognosis	What is the likely course of a patient's illness? What is the balance of the risks and benefits of a treatment?
	Example – cohort study, longitudinal study
Diagnosis	How valid and reliable is a diagnostic test? What does the test tell the doctor?
	Example – cohort study, case-control study
Cost-effectiveness	Which intervention is worth prescribing? Is a newer treatment X worth prescribing compared to an older treatment Y?
	Example – economic analysis
Beliefs, thoughts and experiences	What is it like to live with a disability following a stroke? What is the patient experience of group consultations for learning about the dietary management of diabetes?
	Example – qualitative

Source: Adapted from Burls (1).

Table 7.2 Differences between efficacy and effectiveness studies.

	Efficacy study	Effectiveness study
Question	Does the intervention work under ideal circumstances?	Does the intervention work in real-world practice?
Setting	Resource-intensive 'ideal setting'	Real-world, everyday clinical setting
Study population	Highly selected, homogenous population with several exclusion criteria	Heterogeneous population – few to no exclusion
Providers	Highly experienced and trained	Representative usual providers
Intervention	Strictly enforced and standardised. No concurrent interventions	Applied with flexibility. Concurrent interventions and cross-over permitted

Source: Singal et al. (5)/with permission of Wolters Kluwer Health, Inc.

Box 7.1 **Impact of efficacy and effectiveness**

For detection of hepatocellular carcinoma at an early stage, ultrasound has a sensitivity of 63% in prospective efficacy studies and is regarded as being more efficacious than alpha-fetoprotein. However, in a recent effectiveness study, ultrasound only had a sensitivity of 32%, comparable to that of alpha-fetoprotein (sensitivity 46%) in an effectiveness study. The gap resulted in low utilisation rates of ultrasound and the operator-dependent nature of its diagnostic accuracy.

Source: Singal et al. (22, 23).

---

with early, severe adult respiratory distress syndrome (ARDS). The study reported prolonged prone-positioning ventilation reduced 28-day mortality (HR = 0.39; 95% CI: 0.25–0.63) (3). If the study was well designed and had internal validity, the clinician can assess its transferability to similar patients in the real world. In this example, the results may be applicable to other patients with early, severe ARDS but not to patients with mild ARDS (4). This may limit the external validity of the RCT.

Also important are efficacy and effectiveness. Efficacy is the impact of an intervention under optimal conditions (i.e. trials). Effectiveness determines whether interventions have the intended or expected effects in real clinical settings. Although any given trial may study efficacy more than effectiveness and vice versa, differences between the two exist more on a spectrum than a dichotomy (5). Differences between the two approaches are shown in Table 7.2 (5). Effectiveness research accounts for patient, clinician or organisational factors which may moderate an intervention's implementation in clinical practice (5). Poor access, recommendation, acceptance and adherence rates may result in efficacious interventions being less effective in clinical practice (Box 7.1).

Initial points

Initial points to note about the paper are authors and institutions, including collaborating institutions, the journal and the year of publication. How has the article been peer reviewed? Have the authors made declarations about conflicts of interests, funding and sources of bias? Are there acknowledgements of other contributors?

The journal of publication

Assessing a journal

People are less likely to search for journals specifically. It may be considered as part of critical appraisal once a study of interest has been identified. The impact factor (IF) of a journal is calculated as the number of times its own articles are cited by other articles over a two-year period divided by the total number of articles published by the journal. Citing articles that make up the IF calculation can be from any other journal, including the same journal the original article was published in. For example, the *Annual Review of Vision Science* has an IF of 5.0 (6), meaning that its articles published two years ago will have been cited an average of five times. The IF can suggest the journal's importance in its clinical area, but it should not be used in isolation to assess the quality of an individual article. It is updated annually in June and published in the journal citation report (JCR) (7). The average journal IF is less than 1; 3 is good and 10 remarkable (Table 7.3). Journal citation counts in the JCR include original research, reviews and letters.

Table 7.3 Overview of journal impact factor.

Advantages of publication in a high-impact journal
Increased readership and visibility
Improved academic credibility
Increased grant funding prospects
Improved career advancement
Better validation of research
Increased citations
Higher influence on policymaking
Greater international recognition

Impact factors of well-known journals (2024)	
CA-A Cancer Journal for Clinicians	254.7
Lancet	168.9
New England Journal of Medicine	158.5
Journal of the American Association (JAMA)	120.7
Nature Reviews Drug Discovery	100.3
Nature Reviews Molecular Cell Biology	112.7
British Medical Journal (BMJ)	105.7
Nature Reviews Immunology	100.3
World Psychiatry	73.3
Lancet Psychiatry	64.3

While good articles do get published in journals of lower impact, a high IF indicates a journal is well regarded in its subject area and its articles are likely to be of high quality. The articles have been verified, evaluated, replicated and incorporated into scientific and medical knowledge. Publication in a high-impact journal does not guarantee the quality of any single article, as the IF is applied to the journal and not individual articles.

The title

The title should be clearly written, concise and should convey both the research question and the method of study.

Authorship

To address and provide standards on journal article authorship, the International Committee of Medical Journal Editors stipulates all four of the following criteria for meeting a claim of authorship (8):
1 Substantial contributions to the conception or design of the work or the acquisition, analysis or interpretation of data for the work;
2 Drafting the work or reviewing it critically for important intellectual content;
3 Final approval of the version to be published; and
4 Agreement to be accountable for all aspects of the work in ensuring that questions related to the accuracy or integrity of any part of the work are appropriately investigated and resolved.

Initial questions (9)

1 What is the research question?
2 What is the study design?
3 What are the selection issues?
4 What are the outcome factors, and how are they measured?
5 What are the study factors, and how are they measured?
6 What important confounders are considered?
7 What is the statistical method used in the study?
8 What are the statistical results?
9 What conclusions did the authors reach about the research question?
10 Are ethical issues considered?

The abstract

The abstract should stand alone as an account of the study. Structure will vary from journal to journal but commonly includes: the aims or objectives of the study; the methods including participants, sample size, gender, age and study design (study administration); and outcomes/measurements. Results should describe the main measured variables with statistical analysis and significance. The conclusion should clearly answer the study question.

An abstract will give the 'headlines' for the study, particularly its strengths. It may be less forthcoming about weaknesses in either designs and/or outcomes. Abstract screening for relevance is useful for study selection for further review (e.g. when conducting a systematic review) but should not be relied upon in clinical decision-making. Abstracts should not be used for decision-making at either the individual or population level. Incorporation of a study into a systematic review or clinical guideline always requires the entire article to be fully appraised.

Introduction or background

The introduction provides a context for the study. In quantitative research, this includes review of the known literature, including what is known and remaining gaps. These references should all be listed at the end of the article. A clear explanation of why the new study is required and how it will contribute to knowledge about the topic. The study design and protocol should have been designed prior to any data collection.

Aims and objectives

Most commonly, a study will be used to either test a hypothesis (quantitative research) or generate a hypothesis (qualitative research). This is related to the aim of the study, and it should be clearly stated in the introduction. To avoid bias, the hypothesis should be developed before data collection begins (primary or a priori hypothesis). An explanation should also be given as to why the study is necessary. Reasons could include a gap in existing knowledge, to confirm previous results or to test a new treatment for a condition.

Appraising the study question

The PICO format (PCO format in qualitative studies) can be used to assess the quality of the study question (Chapter 2). The question should be relevant to clinical practice and aim to provide new and meaningful results.

Method

This should describe the study design and why it was chosen. The population studied should be described. Sampling methods should be described, including how the sample was made representative of the population studied. Accounting for sources of bias in study design, sampling and researcher/investigator bias should be identified and an explanation given of how this was minimised in the conduct of the study.

The method should be precise and described clearly so it could be repeated by another investigator. Any interventions studied should be clearly stated. The outcomes to be measured and how they were to be measured, including method of statistical analysis, should be decided upon before the study commences and described clearly in the method.

Although one study should test one hypothesis with one analysis to assess this, it is also common for studies to test further analyses with the study population. This is referred to as subgroup analysis.

A tendency to do multiple subgroup analyses in a single study with subsequent emphasis only on the positive results is referred to as data dredging. Data dredging in multiple subgroups increases the likelihood of positive results being found by chance rather than due to clinically significant differences between study participants. Data dredging may be related to the pressure to get published.

Multiple hypotheses testing in the same study should be avoided, and subgroup analyses should be kept to a minimum. Ideally intended subgroup analyses should be pre-specified in the study protocol (aims and objectives). Where the study data suggests the possibility of an unanticipated subgroup analysis, this should be specified as an exploratory one and not for testing the original hypothesis. The original study question may not be suitable or robust enough for addressing this subsequent subgroup analysis.

The method should confirm ethical approval for the study was sought. The approving committee should be named in the article. Evidence of ethical approval is included in the submission guidelines of journals and will be part of the assessment prior to the paper being sent out for peer review.

Results

This section describes what happened to the participants. This analysis should include or account for all those who dropped out or were lost to follow-up (intention-to-treat analysis). Unanticipated issues with conduct of the study and data collection should be stated. Presentation of results can include raw data with descriptive statistics followed by exploratory and/or confirmatory statistical tests to explain the meaning of the data in relation to the aims and intended outcomes of the study. The reason for the choice of statistical test used should be clear. Data may be explained in both the text and using tables, diagrams and graphs. These should complement, and not repeat, one another. Tables, diagrams and graphs should have clear legends and labelling to aid understanding by the reader.

Discussion/conclusions

This should describe how well the result met the aims of the study and how this fits into the context of existing research. It should also discuss how this may be applied in clinical practice. The inclusion of key points, strengths and limitations, particularly for the clinical context, is helpful in conveying the authors' own understanding of their work as well as providing a summary for the reader. An analysis of how the study findings relate to weakness in the design or the conduct of the study should be included (e.g. intention to treat analysis). General questions in assessing the conclusions include (9):

• Does it consider sources of bias?
• Is the interpretation of the results consistent with the analysed data?
• How is the null hypothesis interpreted?
• Does it relate the study findings to work published previously in this area?
• Are the results generalisable? (external validity)
• Are possible clinical implications and applications described?
• To what are the results, findings and outcomes applicable?
• Does the conclusion answer the study question?
• Is the conclusion credible?
• Are any ethical issues raised by the study?
• Are the results applicable to the patient population for whom you are responsible?
• Can you use this study in your own practice?

Declarations

Journals usually require submitting authors to make several declarations with their article. For published work, these are commonly found at the end of the article. They include whether ethical approval or review was sought, sources of funding and declaration of conflicts of interest.

Conflicts of interest

A conflict of interest arises when the professional judgement of a researcher undertaking a study is affected by a secondary gain from the research. The perception of a conflict of interest is as important as an actual conflict. Any of the researchers may have a conflict of interest, and conflicts may arise at any stage of the study from conception to publication. Conflicts of interest should be declared at the time of ethics approval and submission for publication.

Assessing bias in studies

Bias is the deviation of study findings from the true situation existing within a study population. It can emerge from the question, the study design, methodology, data collection and analysis, presentation of results and conclusions. Different study designs are prone to different forms of bias (Figure 7.1 and Table 7.4). Conducting a study with a preference to reach a particular conclusion, despite evidence to the contrary, is bias.

No study, like any individual or research group, is free from bias. Assessment should focus on what the authors have done to minimise bias during the life of the study, from initial concept to submission for publication. An evaluation should then be made of whether any residual bias in the paper is sufficient to account for the results and whether this invalidates the study. Considering sources at the study design stage can anticipate and avoid bias (Table 7.5) (10).

For intervention studies (RCTs and clinical trials), potential bias leading to differences between the intervention group and non-intervention (control) group should be assessed. The presence of a

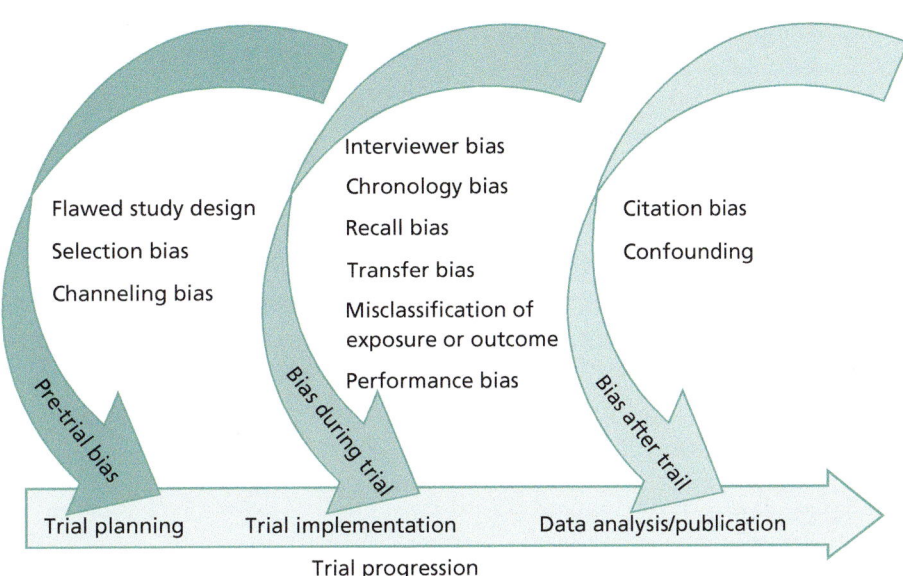

Figure 7.1 Major sources of bias in clinical research. *Source:* Pannucci and Wilkins (10)/with permission of Wolters Kluwer Health, Inc.

Table 7.4 Types of bias in quantitative research.

Bias	Cause
Ascertainment	Some members of a population are more likely to be included than others
Attrition	Systematic bias resulting from those who remain in a study and those who leave it. It can affect analysis of the results
Detection	Systematic differences between groups in how study outcomes are determined
Language	Limiting inclusion of study on basis of language of publication
Performance	The effect of unequal treatment of groups in a study
Publication	The likelihood of a study being published is based on the outcomes of the study – positive results are more likely to be published than negative ones
Randomisation	Randomisation was not properly conducted or properly concealed
Selection	Individuals or groups in a study differ systematically from the population of interest

Source: www.catalogueofbias.org and www.cochrane.org.

Table 7.5 Tips to avoid different types of bias during a trial.

Type of bias	How to avoid
Pre-trial bias	
• Flawed study design	Clearly define risk and outcome, preferably with objective or validated methods. Standardise and blind data collection
• Selection bias	Select patients using rigorous criteria to avoid confounding results. Patients should originate from the same general population. Well-designed prospective studies help to avoid selection bias as the outcome is unknown at the time of enrolment
• Channelling bias	Assign patients to study cohorts using rigorous criteria
Bias during trial	
• Interviewer bias	Standardise the interviewer's interaction with the patient. Blind interviewer to exposure status
• Chronology bias	Prospective studies can eliminate chronology bias
• Recall bias	Use objective data sources whenever possible. When using subjective data sources, corroborate with medical records. Conduct prospective studies because the outcome is unknown at the time of patient enrolment
• Transfer bias	Carefully design the study plan for lost-to-follow-up patients prior to the study
• Exposure misclassification	Clearly define exposure prior to the study. Avoid using proxies of exposure
• Outcome misclassification	Use objective diagnostic studies or validated measures as primary outcome
• Performance bias	Consider cluster stratification to minimise variability technique
Bias after trial	
• Citation bias	Register a trial with an accepted clinical trials registry. Check registries for similar unpublished or in-progress trials prior to publication
• Confounding	Known confounders can be controlled with study design (case-control design or randomisation) or during data analysis (regression). Unknown confounders can only be controlled with randomisation

Source: Pannucci and Wilkins (10)/with permission of Wolters Kluwer Health, Inc.

comparison group where any intervention study is undertaken is a controlled trial. Intervention and control groups should be similar for all characteristics except for the intervention being tested. If one group has a significantly different frequency of characteristic (e.g. age, gender identity and weight), this may prove to be the explanation for any observed difference. Where trials are randomised, the randomisation should be clearly explained, including if concealed allocation was used and whether the patients and investigators were blinded to the treatment being given to arms of the trial.

Inclusion in subgroup analysis

A challenge for evidence-based healthcare is improvement of inclusion in healthcare (Chapter 9). Historically, groups including ethnic minorities and women have been under-represented in clinical research. Even in large trials, subgroups of underserved and minoritised groups may not be large enough for valid analysis. This has an impact on assessing the application of research findings to minoritised groups.

Reporting standards

Reporting standards for studies were discussed in Chapter 4. The EQUATOR Network (11) recommends guidelines for each type of study design. Since its establishment in 2006, EQUATOR has promoted accurate and transparent reporting of research through its dissemination of recommended guidelines. It is essential that researchers understand the study design they are using so it is reported using the appropriate guidelines. Preparation of a manuscript for publication should use both the appropriate study reporting guideline and the journal-specific guidance for authors (12).

Assessment of the quality of evidence reported in a journal article is the role of critical appraisal. Reporting guidelines provide authors with minimum standards for publishing the results of their research. A poorly reported study is likely to receive a poor critical appraisal. Consequently, it is less likely to be considered for wider dissemination and synthesis in systematic reviews and meta-analyses (12).

Appraisal tools

Critical appraisal tools provide a structured worksheet to assist the assessment of the reliability, quality, importance and wider application of published evidence in clinical practice.

The critical appraisal skills programme (CASP) (13)

This programme, developed initially by the University of Oxford, UK, exists to help people develop critical appraisal skills. The programme has produced checklists to assist the appraisal of the validity, results and relevance of different study designs (Box 7.2). These are open access and can be downloaded free of charge from the CASP website (see Further Resources). The CASP checklists cover study validity, results and clinical relevance. The first two

---

Box 7.2 Critical appraisal skills programme checklists

- Systematic reviews with meta-analysis of observational studies
- Systematic reviews with meta-analysis of randomised controlled trials (RCTs)
- Randomised controlled trial (RCT) checklist
- Systematic review checklist
- Qualitative studies checklist
- Cohort study checklist
- Diagnostic study checklist
- Case-control study checklist
- Economic evaluation checklist
- Clinical prediction rule checklist

Source: Adapted from https://casp-uk.net/casp-tools-checklists/, last accessed on 17 September 2024.

Table 7.6 Examples of widely used research reporting guidelines.

Study design	Reporting guidelines
Systematic reviews/meta-analyses	PRISMA
Meta-analysis of observation studies in epidemiology	MOOSE
Synthesis of qualitative research	ENTREQ
Randomised trials	CONSORT
Intervention evaluation studies using non-randomised designs	TREND
Cohort, case-control and cross-sectional studies	STROBE
Case report	CARE
Web-based surveys	CHERRIES
Qualitative research	COREQ
Mixed-methods studies	GAMMS
Economic evaluations of interventions	CHEERS
Systematic review and meta-analysis protocols	PRISMA-P
Diagnostic accuracy studies	STARD
Development, validation or update of a prediction model	TRIPOD

Source: Haile (12)/with permission of SAGE Publications.

---

questions in each checklist are screening questions. If the user cannot answer 'Yes' to these questions, the article is unlikely to be helpful and should be disregarded. In addition to the checklists, CASP also provides training in their use and critical appraisal more generally.

Other tools are the Cochrane risk of bias tool used in assessment of RCTs, the Joanna Briggs Institute (JBI) tool and the evaluation tool for qualitative studies (ETQS). CASP is well established and familiar. The ETQS provides more detail than CASP on how to interpret criteria in qualitative studies. However, a comparison of three tools found the JBI tool to be most coherent in its approach to qualitative research (see Chapter 5) (14). Tables 7.6 and 7.7 show further examples and applications of reporting standards and appraisal tools (12). The tools can be downloaded and printed. They are structured and facilitate critical appraisal for both novices and experts.

Table 7.7 Examples of commonly used appraisal tools.

Tool	Authors/organisation
Critical appraisal skills programme (CASP)	CASP
Appraisal of guidelines for research and evaluation II (AGREE II)	AGREE collaboration
John Hopkins research evidence appraisal tool John Hopkins non-research evidence appraisal tool	The John Hopkins Hospital and University
Grading of recommendations assessment, Development and evaluation (GRADE)	GRADE working group
Cochrane risk of bias tool	Cochrane collaboration
Joanna Briggs Institute critical appraisal tools (JBI)	Joanna Briggs Institute
Rapid critical appraisal checklists	Melnyk and Fineout-Overholt
Centre for Evidence-Based Medicine critical appraisal tools (CEBM)	The Oxford Centre for Evidence-Based Medicine
A measurement tool to assess systematic reviews 2 (AMSTAR 2)	Shea et al. (15)
Quality assessment of diagnostic accuracy studies 2 (QUADAS 2)	Whiting et al. (16)

Source: Haile (12)/with permission of SAGE Publications.

Systematic reviews and meta-analyses

Systematic reviews are the most widely used form of evidence synthesis. They attempt to review and, where possible, combine the results of studies. These can be either primary studies at the base of the evidence pyramid (Chapter 3) or RCTs. Evidence is selected based on the review question, inclusion and exclusion criteria and the similarity of the methodology of studies identified in the evidence search. The QUADAS-2 tool facilitates critical appraisal of systematic reviews (17). When selecting evidence for a systematic review, the evidence can be selected using the grading recommendations of assessment, development and evaluation (GRADE) (18). Selection of evidence is an essential step, and grading it helps to formulate the recommendations arising from the review. Evidence is graded on a four-point scale – very low, low, moderate or high. Experimental studies are likely to be graded as high and observational studies as low or very low.

Meta-analyses

A meta-analysis is where the results of several studies have been combined to create a larger sample. This pooling of results from several studies provides greater statistical power for the recommendations of the analysis. It enables calculation of the effect size and magnitude of an intervention. Meta-analyses are often used to combine the results of RCTs. The quality of the analysis is dependent on the quality of the original RCTs. The method is susceptible to publication bias. Funnel plots are used to estimate the effects of publication bias in a meta-analysis (Figure 7.2).

An important concept in combination of results in a meta-analysis is heterogeneity. This term reflects the differences in the

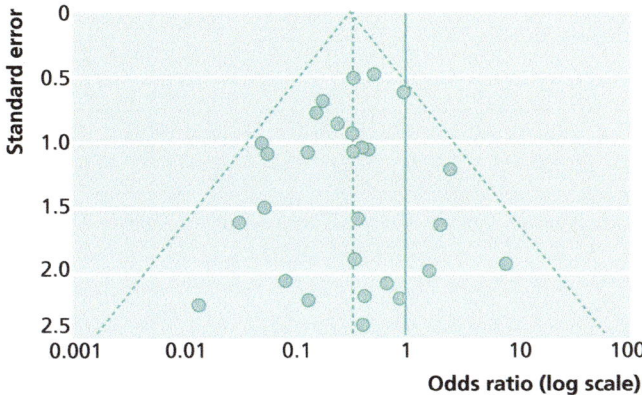

Figure 7.2 Explanation of a funnel plot. The outer dashed lines indicate the triangular region within which 95% of the studies are expected to lie in the absence of both biases and heterogeneity (fixed effect summary log odds ratio ±1.96 × standard error of summary log odds ratio). The solid vertical line corresponds to no intervention effect. *Source:* Sterne et al. (19)/with permission of BMJ Publishing Group Ltd.

estimates of effects of the studies selected for the meta-analysis. Even with the same intervention, differences between studies arise due to differences in the population investigated in each study, the study protocol, how it was conducted and sources of bias. Heterogeneity of studies selected for meta-analysis can be analysed statistically (I^2 test). Values for heterogeneity are low (0–40%), moderate (30–60%), substantial (50–90%) and considerable (75–100%). Heterogeneity is present where I^2 is greater than 50%. Where studies are similar (homogeneous), these can be combined in a subgroup analysis with the effect of an intervention being compared between the identified subgroups.

Homogeneous studies can be combined in a 'fixed effects model' where it is assumed there is one true effect and it is the same across all the studies selected. Where there is heterogeneity across studies, the differences between studies are assumed to be true, and a mean value for the studies and estimation of effect size is calculated. Use of a forest plot allows the similarities and differences between studies in a meta-analysis to be visualised (Figure 7.3).

The six basic columns of a forest plot are: included studies, intervention group, control group, weighting of each study as a proportion of the total number of participants, outcome measure in numerical form and outcome measure in graphical form. The solid vertical line in the graph represents the 'line of no effect'. In Figure 8.7, the studies and the summary 'diamond' lie to the right of the line of no effect. The meta-analysis has demonstrated the intervention across the four studies included is statistically significant. Critical appraisal of the statistical calculations in a study is crucial in determining its quality and strength of evidence.

Acknowledgements

Thank you to Alistair Hewins, a final year graduate entry medicine student at the University of Nottingham, UK, for his contribution to the journal impact factor of this chapter.

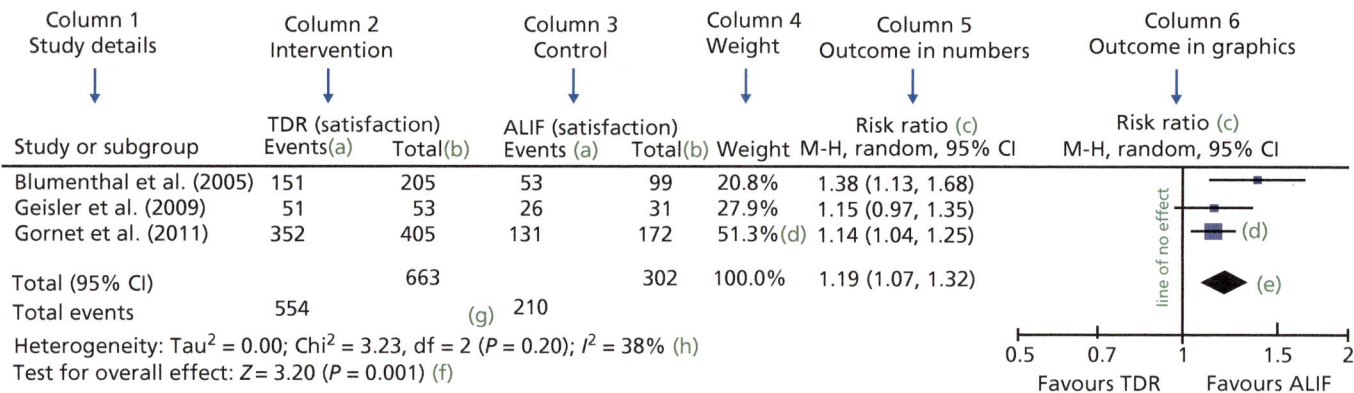

(a) Number of events
(b) Populations size (sample size)
(c) Risk ratio in numeric and graphical presentation
(d) Size of the box represents study weight
(e) Pooled effect and 95% CI does not cross the line of no effect
(f) $P = 0.001$ (test for overall effect) confirms statistical significance illustrated by the diamond not crossing the line of effect
(g) $P = 0.20$, we do not reject the hypothesis of no heterogeneity
(h) Amount of heterogeneity might not be important (<40%)

Figure 7.3 Example of a forest plot from a meta-analysis. Proportion of patients satisfied with total disc replacement (TDR) versus anterior lumbar interbody fusion (ALIF). *Source:* Mu et al. (20), Dettori et al. (21)/JMIR Publications/CC BY 4.0.

References

1 Burls, A. (2014). *What is Critical Appraisal?* Newmarket: Hayward Medical Communications.

2 Akobeng, A.K. (2008). Assessing the validity of clinical trials. *J Pediatr Gastroenterol Nutr* 47 (3): 277–282.

3 Guérin, C., Reignier, J., Richard, J.C. et al. (2013). Prone positioning in severe acute respiratory distress syndrome. *N Engl J Med* 368 (23): 2159–2168.

4 Patino, C.M. and Ferreira, J.C. (2018). Internal and external validity: can you apply research study results to your patients? *J Bras Pneumol* 44 (3): 183.

5 Singal, A.G., Higgins, P.D., and Waljee, A.K. (2014). A primer on effectiveness and efficacy trials. *Clin Transl Gastroenterol* 5 (1): e45.

6 Annual Reviews (2015). Annual review of vision science Published since 2015. https://www.annualreviews.org/content/journals/vision (accessed 20 November 2024).

7 Clarivate, Academia & Government (2024). Journal citation reports. https://clarivate.com/products/scientific-and-academic-research/research-analytics-evaluation-and-management-solutions/journal-citation-reports/ (accessed 20 November 2024).

8 ICoMJ (2024). Up-dated ICMJE recommendations. https://www.icmje.org/news-and-editorials/updated_recommendations_jan2024.html (accessed 20 November 2024).

9 Al-Jundi, A. and Sakka, S. (2017). Critical appraisal of clinical research. *J Clin Diagn Res* 11 (5): Je01–Je05.

10 Pannucci, C.J. and Wilkins, E.G. (2010). Identifying and avoiding bias in research. *Plast Reconstr Surg* 126 (2): 619–625.

11 (2006) Equator network. https://www.equator-network.org (accessed 20 November 2022).

12 Haile, Z.T. (2022). Critical appraisal tools and reporting guidelines. *J Hum Lact* 38 (1): 21–27.

13 Critical Appraisal Skills Programme (2023). CASP checklists. https://casp-uk.net (accessed 20 November 2024).

14 Hannes, K., Lockwood, C., and Pearson, A. (2010). A comparative analysis of three online appraisal instruments' ability to assess validity in qualitative research. *Qual Health Res* 20 (12): 1736–1743.

15 Shea, B.J., Reeves, B.C., Wells, G. et al. (2017). AMSTAR 2: a critical appraisal tool for systematic reviews that include randomised or non-randomised studies of healthcare interventions, or both. *BMJ* 358: j4008.

16 Whiting, P.F., Rutjes, A.W., Westwood, M.E. et al. (2011). QUADAS-2: a revised tool for the quality assessment of diagnostic accuracy studies. *Ann Intern Med* 155 (8): 529–536.

17 QUADAS-2. https://www.bristol.ac.uk/media-library/sites/quadas/migrated/documents/quadas2.pdf (accessed 20 November 2024).

18 Grade. https://www.gradeworkinggroup.org (accessed 20 November 2024).

19 Sterne, J.A., Sutton, A.J., Ioannidis, J.P. et al. (2011). Recommendations for examining and interpreting funnel plot asymmetry in meta-analyses of randomised controlled trials. *BMJ* 22 (343): d4002. https://doi.org/10.1136/bmj.d4002. PMID: 21784880.

20 Mu, X., Wei, J., Jiancuo, A. et al. (2018). The short-term efficacy and safety of artificial total disc replacement for selected patients with lumbar degenerative disc disease compared with anterior lumbar interbody fusion: a systematic review and meta-analysis. *PLoS One* 13 (12): e0209660. https://doi.org/10.1371/journal.pone.0209660. PMID: 30592739; PMCID: PMC6310255.

21 Dettori, J.R., Norvell, D.C., and Chapman, J.R. (2021). Seeing the forest by looking at the trees: how to interpret a meta-analysis forest plot. *Global Spine J* 11 (4): 614–616. https://doi.org/10.1177/21925682211003889. PMID: 33939533; PMCID: PMC8119923.

22 Singal, A.G., Yopp, A.S., Skinner, C. et al. (2012). Utilization of hepatocellular carcinoma surveillance among American patients: a systematic review. *J Gen Intern Med* 27 (7): 861–867.

23 Singal, A.G., Conjeevaram, H.S., Volk, M.L. et al. (2012). Effectiveness of hepatocellular carcinoma surveillance in patients with cirrhosis. *Cancer Epidemiol Biomarkers Prev* 21 (5): 793–799.

Further reading

Gosall, N. and Gosall, G. (2015). *The Doctor's Guide to Critical Appraisal*, 4e. Knutsford: Pastest.

Greenhalgh, T. (2019). *How to Read a Paper: The Basics of Evidence-Based Medicine and Healthcare*, 6e. Oxford: Wiley.

CHAPTER 8

Evidence into Practice

John Frain

Division of Medical Sciences and Graduate Entry Medicine, University of Nottingham, Nottingham, UK

OVERVIEW

- To benefit patients, evidence must be translated into real-world practice.
- Implementation science establishes whether and how research should be applied in practice.
- Implementation science analyses the facilitators and barriers to translation of evidence into practice by healthcare providers and professionals.
- The evidence for diagnoses and therapies should be explained to patients through shared decision-making.
- Shared decision-making and communication of risk to patients require clinical communication and reasoning skills.
- Statistical concepts of risk are often poorly understood by patients and clinicians.

Introduction

While statistical tests establish the statistical significance of a difference between groups in, for example, an RCT (randomised controlled trial) and not due to chance, this alone does not mean the result is suitable for application in clinical practice. Clinical significance differs from statistical significance in considering the practical relevance and importance of research results. To be clinically significant, the observed difference between, for example, an intervention and control group in an RCT also has to have an impact on patient care and outcomes. Clinically significant research is statistically rigorous and clinically relevant. Clinically relevant research also needs to take account of patient preferences and values. Though individuals and teams may be able to make some of these decisions, the volume and breadth of research published means this usually requires the work of many individuals and approaches at an organisational, local, national or international level.

Patient and public involvement

Ensuring research benefits patients and is facilitated by their involvement at several levels. Public engagement helps to disseminate research findings and increase awareness of research priorities for patients, the public and professionals. Increasing researcher awareness of what matters to patients is related to research quality and impact. Funding is now often dependent on evidence of PPI. Patients and the public are increasingly involved in reviewing research proposals, on research commissioning panels and as co-applicants for research projects. UK Standards for Public Involvement in Research provide a framework covering:

- Opportunities to be involved in research groups
- Contributing to productive and mutually respectful relationships
- Providing learning and support for building skills for public involvement in research
- Developing plain language resources to explain and promote research topics
- Empowering the public by sharing the achievements of public involvement in research
- Involving the public in management, regulation, leadership and decision-making in research programmes

Knowledge-to-action cycle

The knowledge-to-action cycle provides a model for selecting implementation strategies. The model centres on the initial research and the need to synthesise evidence. It provides outline recommendations for steps to effect policies for change. These comprise both knowledge and action. The cyclical nature of the model reflects the continuous nature of evidence translation and implementation (Figure 8.1) (1).

Often clinicians lack the time, expertise and resources to implement research in clinical practice. There can be a long interval between publication of research and its adoption into practice, often years or decades (2).

Implementation science

Implementation science addresses this problem by building knowledge about how evidence is adopted, factors causing delay and those facilitating accelerated and successful implementation of evidence into practice. By facilitating translation of evidence into practice, implementation science can improve patient care and outcomes (3). However, widespread change is difficult to achieve (4).

ABC of Evidence-Based Healthcare, First Edition. Edited by John Frain.
© 2025 John Frain. Published 2025 by John Wiley & Sons Ltd.

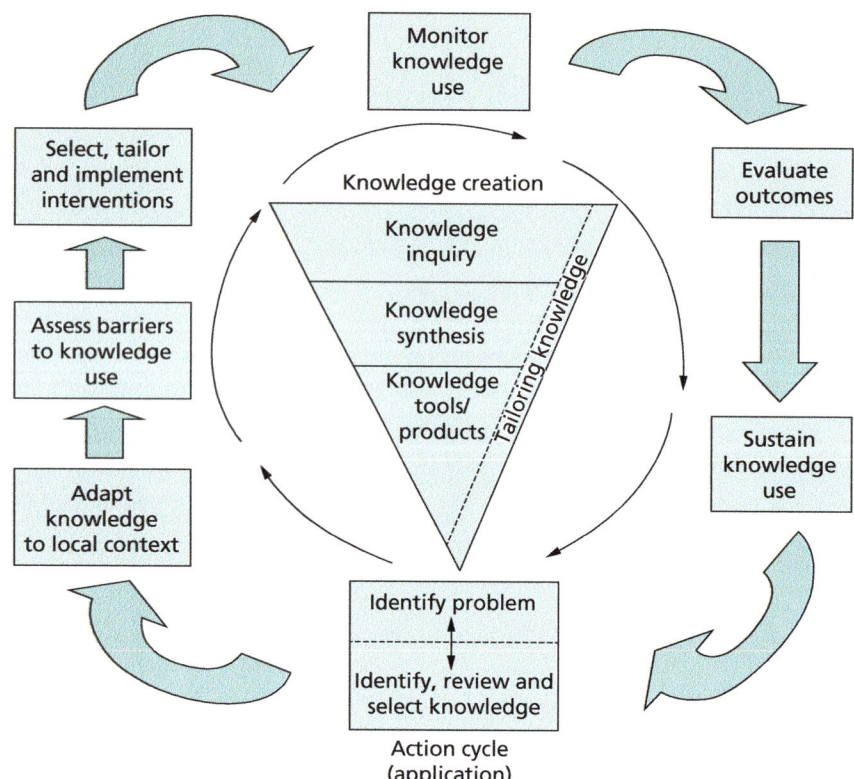

Figure 8.1 Knowledge-to-action cycle. *Source:* Straus (1)/with permission of BMJ Publishing Group Ltd.

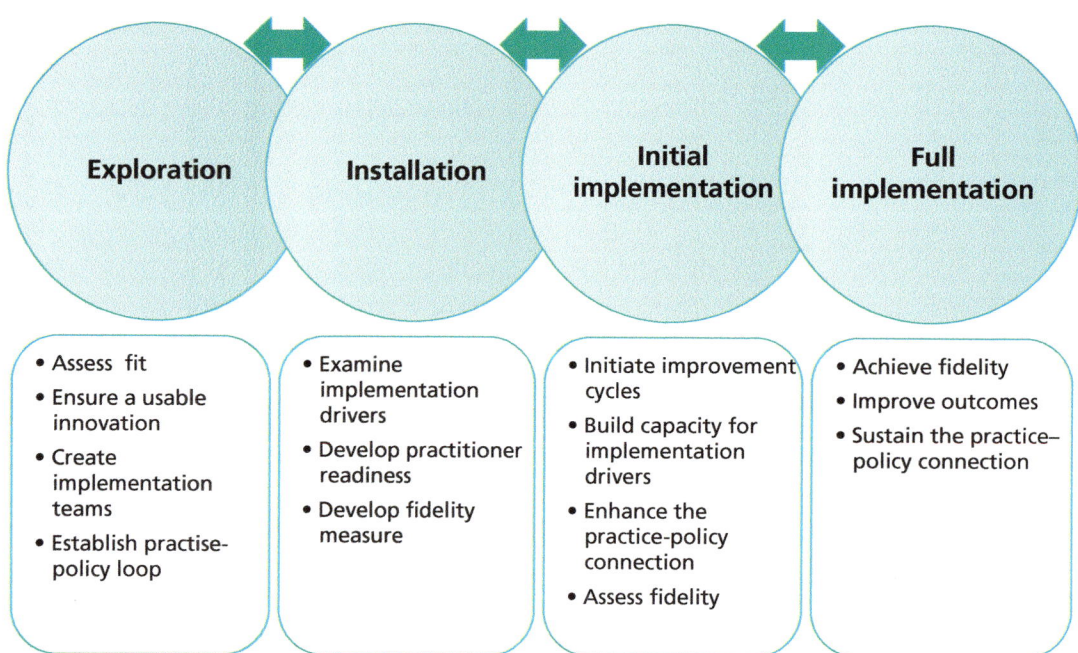

Figure 8.2 Use of the active implementation framework for a community-based mental health intervention for child health in the Amazon. *Source:* Westgard and Fleming (7)/JMIR Publications/CC BY 4.0.

Small, low-level changes successful in one setting may be the opposite in others (5). Implementation science provides a structured and phased approach to implementation in multiple sites (4). Approaches include the social sciences which examine the contextual factors in which organisations and individuals must implement evidence into practice (4).

Implementation science tools provide a structured approach to all phases of the cycle (6). An example is the Active Implementation Framework (Figure 8.2) (7). This comprises five distinct frameworks: (i) usable innovations, (ii) implementation stages, (iii) implementation drivers, (iv) implementation teams and (v) improvement cycles.

Guidelines

The achievements of evidence-based healthcare include the development of systematic review methodology. The 1990s saw not only the beginning of evidence-based healthcare but also the proliferation of guidelines across all healthcare professions and specialties. Clinical guidelines are underpinned by a systematic review of the evidence, including an assessment of bias. A guideline development group will assess the quality of the evidence. Relevant stakeholders, such as representatives of relevant health professions, health organisations and patients, should be included in consultation prior to the guideline publication. While a guideline should be introduced only where it is likely to have a positive impact on clinical outcomes for patients, the recommendations in any new guideline, though themselves evidence-based, will not necessarily have been validated. This should be done prospectively, and the guideline should be updated as the evidence changes. The circumstances in which the guideline should be used and the patients to whom it applies should be clearly stated. Where there are several guidelines for the same or similar conditions, there may be differences in the recommendations. Clinical judgement should still be applied to the appropriate use of a guideline in the individual patient. Good guidelines also account for the cost-effectiveness of its implementation. Guidelines may be more difficult to apply in patients with more than one, particularly, chronic condition. Improving adoption and adherence to clinical guidelines remains a challenge for evidence-based healthcare (Chapter 9) (8).

Clinical reasoning, evidence, communication and shared decision-making

Shared decision-making is a component of clinical reasoning (Figure 8.3) (9). It is also incorporated into evidence-based models of clinical communication where the explanation skills required include providing the correct type and amount of information, aiding accurate recall and understanding and incorporating the patient's illness framework (Figure 8.4).

Shared decision-making builds upon Sackett's definition of evidence-based medicine (Sackett 1996) and is defined as (12):

'An approach where clinicians and patients make decisions together using the best available evidence. Patients are encouraged to think about the available screening, treatment, or management options and the likely benefit and harms of each so that they can communicate their preferences and help select the best course of action for them. Shared decision-making respects patient autonomy and promotes patient engagement'

Shared decision-making requires understanding of the preferences and values of others. This means inclusive communication and history taking together with cultural humility (Chapter 9). For the patient, shared decision-making requires understanding of the harms and benefits of healthcare options, including diagnostic and treatment procedures. This requires patient health literacy and adequate risk communication by the clinician (13, 14).

'Evidence-based medicine needs shared decision making, and shared decision-making needs evidence-based medicine. Patients need both' (15). Effective sharing of decision-making by clinicians requires access to evidence, time to assimilate it and the clinical communication training to discuss it clearly with patients. There are facilitators and barriers to this (Figure 8.5) (16). Models of shared decision-making have been described (Figure 8.6) (13). Key phases in the discussion are:

- Active listening
- Access to high-quality evidence
- Providing information tailored to the individual patient
- Aiding accurate recall and understanding
- Encouraging and answering questions
- Achieving a shared understanding
- The patient plays an active role in the decision
- Agreeing a decision (including deferral of the decision)

Though evidence-based healthcare and shared decision-making are interdependent, they are rarely taught alongside one another (Chapter 10). Much teaching of evidence-based healthcare concentrates on the first three steps (ask, acquire and appraise) and not 'apply' or 'evaluate'. Consequently, the most

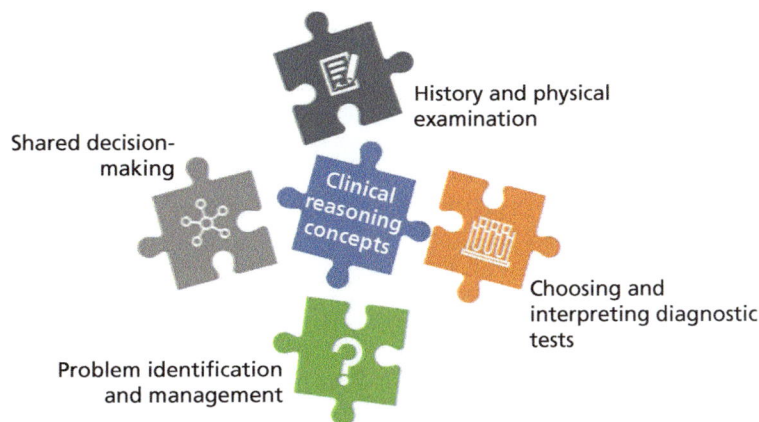

Figure 8.3 Five broad areas of clinical reasoning education. *Source:* Cooper et al. (9)/John Wiley & Sons. Clinical reasoning concepts include key theories (e.g. script and dual process), how clinical reasoning ability develops, the problem of diagnostic error, the role of clinical reasoning in safe and effective care for patients, cognitive errors and other factors that may impair the clinical reasoning process or outcome. *Source:* Cooper and Frain (10)/John Wiley & Sons.

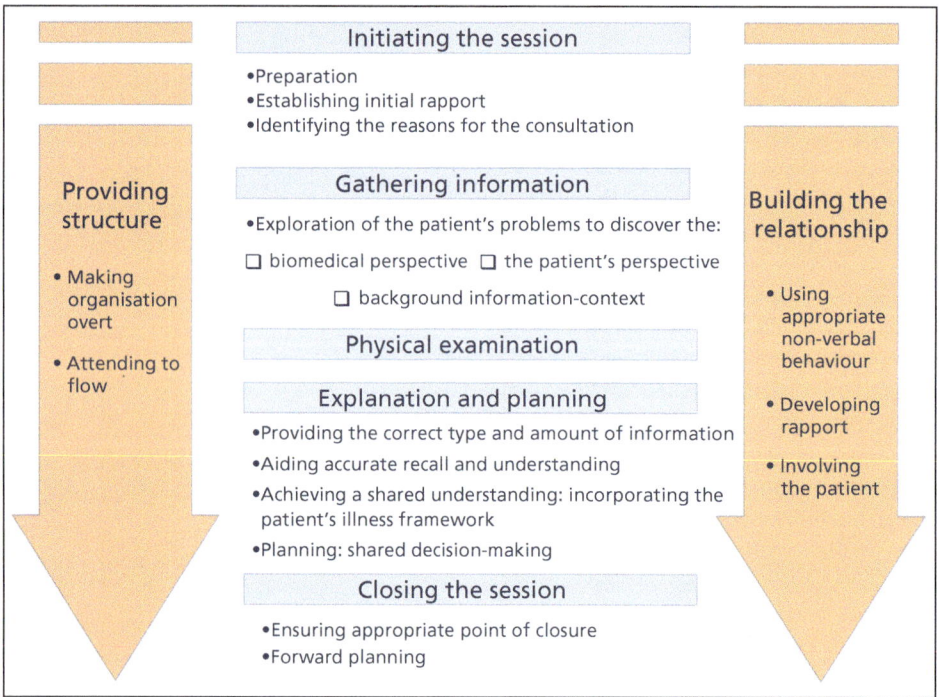

Figure 8.4 The Calgary Cambridge Guide – the expanded framework. *Source:* Silverman (11)/John Wiley & Sons.

Combining evidence and patient preferences

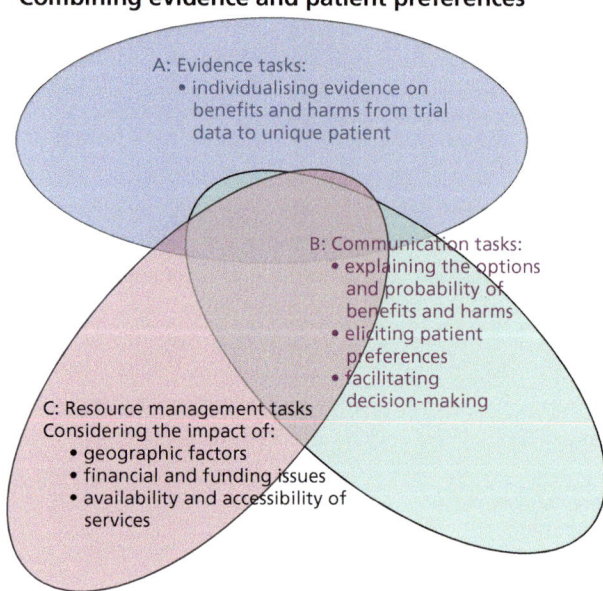

Figure 8.5 Evidence-based healthcare and shared decision-making. *Source:* Barratt (16)/with permission of Elsevier.

frequently cited barriers to shared decision-making are lack of formal training, lack of shared decision making (SDM) skills and knowledge and uncertainty about the situations in which to use shared decision-making (16). Some clinicians worry it will add time to patient consultations when this is in fact minimal (17).

Patient health literacy

One in three to almost one in two Europeans (27–48%) have problems in comprehending and using health information (18). Similar rates are reported in Canada (19). Limited health literacy (LHL) is associated with lower socio-economic background, migrant background, limited education and chronic conditions (20). However, LDL may occur in highly educated people. Associations with limited health literacy (LDL) are shown in Box 8.1. Involving patients with LDL in shared decision-making improves patient participation, increases knowledge, informed choice, self-efficacy and reduces conflict in decision-making (20). Accounting for a patient's level of health literacy is especially important in the initial phase of shared decision-making – choice talk.

Clear communication is essential in option talk and risk communication. However, the terminology used to describe risk is heterogeneous, making it difficult for patients to understand what is being described. Examples include 'risk', 'probability', 'chance' and 'likelihood' are used interchangeably even though they have different meanings from one another (20). Describing the 'probability of benefits and harms' is recommended as the most appropriate term for communicating risk within shared decision-making (14).

Communicating risk to patients

Risk communication strategies are intended to convey to patients the numerical probabilities of the benefits and harms of health options (Figure 8.7) (20). Risk communication is a core element of option

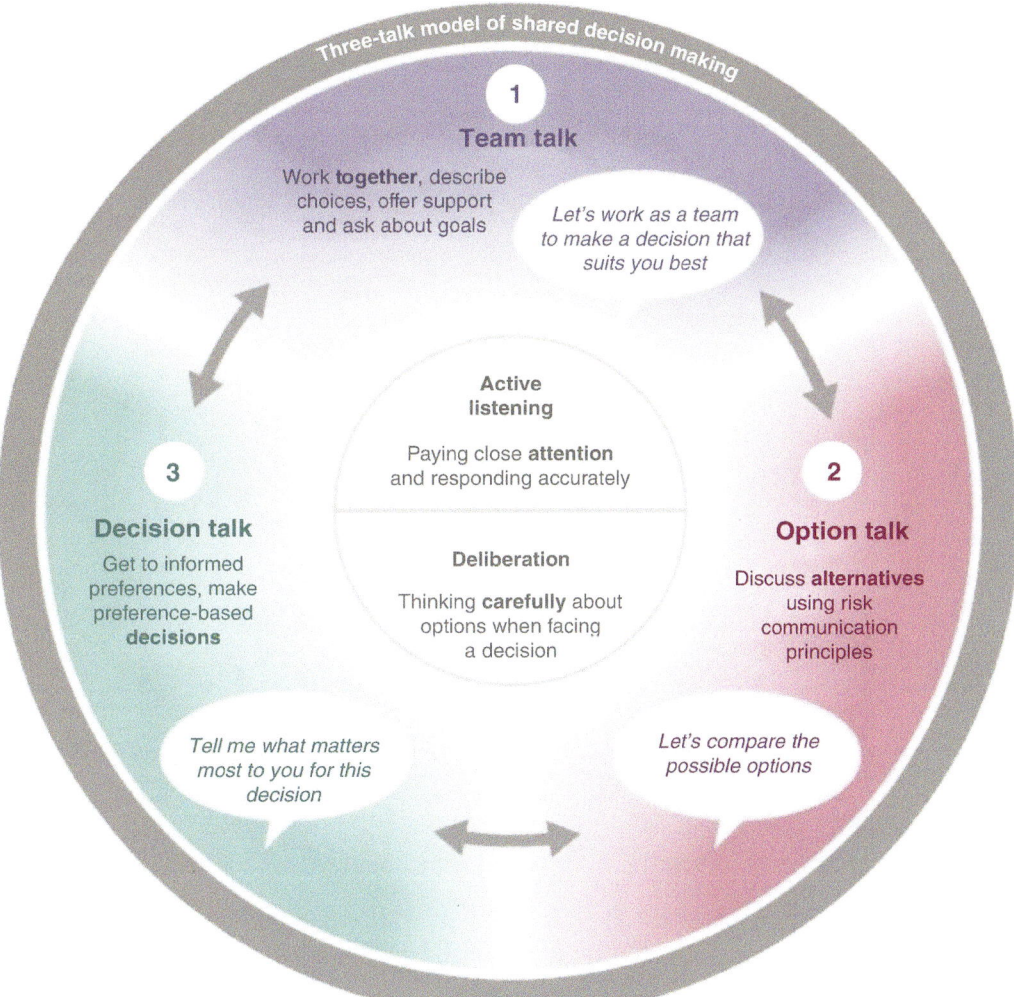

Figure 8.6 Three-talk model of shared decision-making. *Source:* Elwyn et al. (13)/with permission of BMJ Publishing Group Ltd.

Box 8.1 **Associations with low health literacy in adults**

- Poorer understanding of medical information, medical conditions and related care
- Struggle to use medication correctly
- Management of chronic diseases is poorer
- Patients make riskier health choices – e.g. smoking
- Poorer adherence to medication
- Impairments in the process and use of information
  - Aspects of numeracy
    - Understanding of probabilistic treatment information
  - Graph literacy skills

Source: Richter (20)/with permission of Elsevier.

communication is a strategy for risk management. It leads to better understanding by both parties and better clinical decision-making.

Framing of information refers to providing information, numerically or verbally, in different ways. Positive and negative framing are commonly used strategies and are used to describe the chance of survival (positive) or chance of death (negative) (19). Positive framing is more likely to be effective for explanation and acceptance of the risk of high-risk procedures such as surgery, though this may also be influenced by clinician bias.

Decision aids

Trials of patient decision aids (PDAs) and tools including question prompt list show good effects in risk communication (Box 8.2) (2). PDAs provide evidence-based information about therapeutic options and associated benefits and harms. A Cochrane systematic review updated on three occasions has consistently found large increases in patient knowledge, accurate risk perceptions and an active role in decision-making (17). There is less decision regret, and patients report feeling informed and clear about personal values.

talk during shared decision-making. Where information is provided about the likely probability of an outcome, the accuracy of a patient's risk perception improves (21). Otherwise, many patients tend to under- or overestimate their risk with impact on choices. Risk

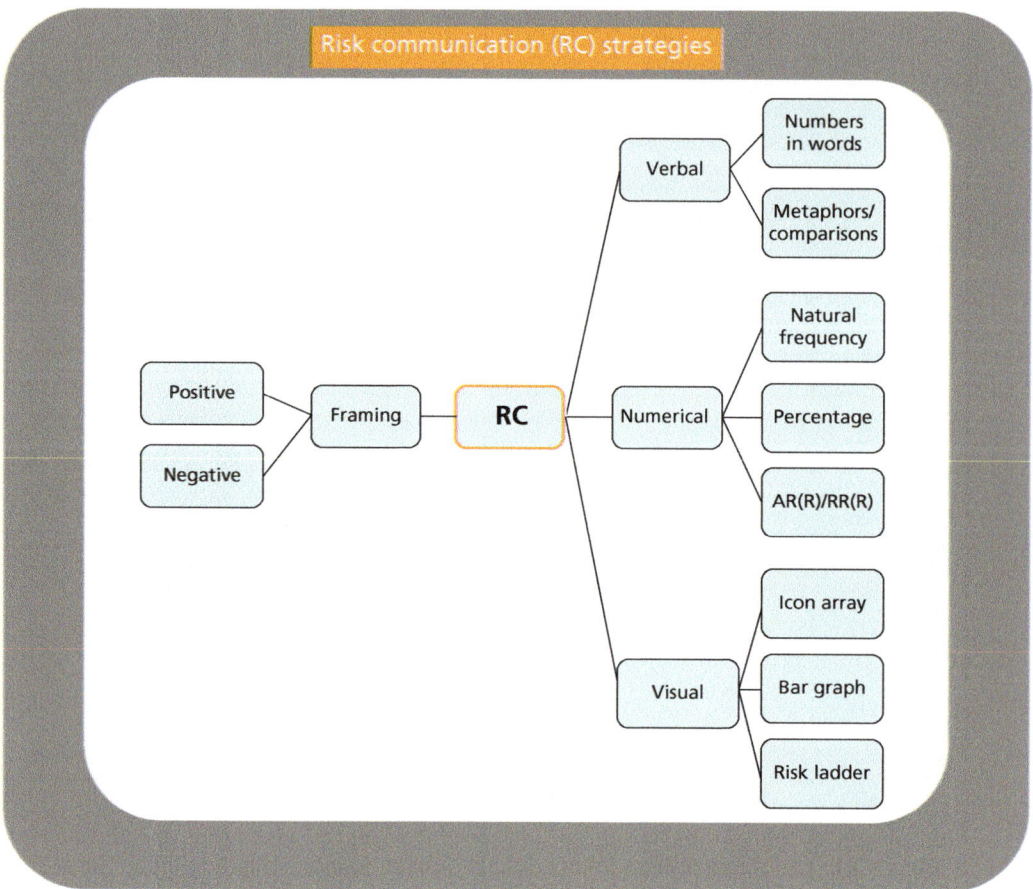

Figure 8.7 Overview of risk communication strategies. *Source:* Richter et al. (20)/with permission of Elsevier.

Box 8.2 **Strategies for risk communication during option talk**

- Consider the cognitive load of the discussion on your patient
- Use descriptive frequencies (e.g. 1 in 10 or 1 in 100) or percentages
- Use a well-defined denominator explaining who the risk is about and over what time period (e.g. 4 in 1000 men aged 60 will die from prostate cancer over the next 10 years)
- Use a consistent denominator (e.g. '1 in 1000 and 30 in 1000' not '1 in 40 and 1 in 250')
- Avoid purely descriptive terms (e.g. low risk, moderate risk and high risk)
- Risk should be quantified as absolute rather than relative risk
- Balanced framing (i.e. chances of survival and chances of death)
- Serious harm should be described, however unlikely
- Use appropriate visual aids, such as pictographs or icon arrays
- Patient understanding can be checked using 'chunking and checking' and 'teach back' methods
- Share uncertainty if and when the best decision is genuinely unclear

Source: Adapted from Edwards (26).

Visual aids

Use of visual aids alongside numerical information improves accuracy and comprehension of risk by both patients and clinicians. Information is better understood where 'healthy' and 'sick' patients appear together in the schematic. Examples of decision aids can be seen in Figures 8.8 and 8.9. Further examples of decision aids include 'Wiser Choices' in the United States and Option Grids in the United Kingdom (see useful websites). Wiser Choices PDAs provide visual information which combines both evidence and patient values. For example, a decision aid on antidepressants combines information on 'what you need to know', weight change, sexual issues, sleep, cost, stopping and side effects. Option grids are intended to provide one-page summaries answering patients' frequent questions (23). This can be used as the basis for a structured and comprehensive discussion.

Statistical concepts

We have kept the statistics of risk until now so it can be considered alongside clinical reasoning, communication and shared decision-making. Clinicians also report difficulty in

Over the next 5 years

88
people will have
no stroke

4
people will have
a fatal or
disabling stroke

8
people will have
a non-disabling
stroke

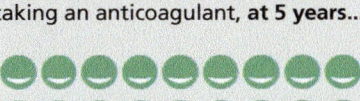

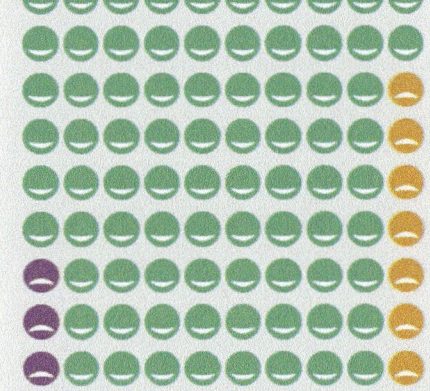

Current
Risk of stroke
without anticoagulation

In 100 people like you who **are not**
taking an anticoagulant, **at 5 years...**

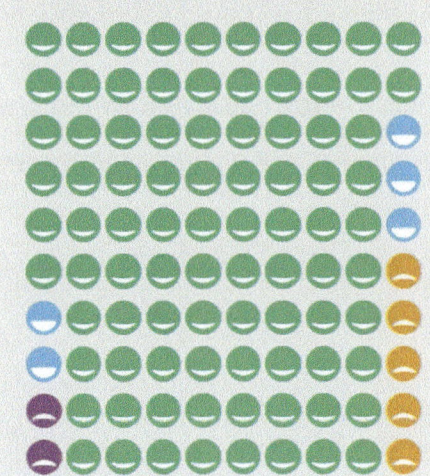

Future
Risk of stroke
with anticoagulation

In 100 people like you who **are** taking
an anticoagulant, **at 5 years...**

Over the next 5 years

93
people will have
no stroke

2
people will have
a fatal or
disabling stroke

5
people will have
a non-disabling
stroke

5
people will
avoid a stroke
by taking
anticoagulation

The risk of stroke, with and without anticoagulation, are depicted using a visual representation of 100 patients, each with similar stroke risk based on CHA2DS2-VASc score. A representative proportion of this population who would be expected to have either a fatal/disabling stroke or a non-disabling stroke are colored in yellow or purple. Individuals who would be spared an anticipated stroke with anticoagulation are colored in blue

Figure 8.8 Patient decision aid (PDA) for use of anticoagulation in the prevention of stroke in patients with atrial fibrillation. *Source:* Noseworthy et al. (22)/ with permission of Springer Nature.

understanding the meaning of statistical measurements of risk. A survey across eight countries among doctors in various specialities and of varying levels of experience found that most had difficulty understanding measures of magnitude such as relative risk (RR) (24). There are also reported difficulties in understanding the concepts of risk and probability (19). Despite increased training in healthcare curricula, levels of statistical literacy among clinicians appear not to have increased over the past 40 years (19).

The commonly required statistical measures of risk are as displayed in Table 8.1 (19). In communicating risk to patients, clinicians should consider which is the most appropriate measure of the risk they are wishing to convey to the patient, whether they themselves can comfortably explain it and how well the patient is likely to receive the information particularly where there is low health literacy. Natural frequencies supported by decision aids are the measures of magnitude or effect size most easily understood (e.g. 1000-person diagrams) (19). The decision-making with the patient should be discussed and recorded in the record. It may be appropriate to provide the patient with a PDA or link to one and allow time for the patient to reflect and/or discuss with family members before they make a decision (Box 8.3).

Relative risk versus absolute risk

The size of the number presented to the patient may affect how risk is perceived by the patient. A study examining the acceptance or decline of a hypothetical treatment to prevent hip fractures found patients more likely to accept the treatment when benefits were presented in absolute terms. Box 8.4 illustrates a study of risk communication for a screening test where the identical benefits were presented in terms of absolute risk reduction (ARR), relative risk reduction (RRR) or numbers needed to treat (NNT) (25). Patients were more likely to take the test when the risk was presented as RRR and least likely when presented as NNT. Clinicians must be clear at the outset about how statistical information needs to be presented to facilitate the patient making an informed decision. Patients should be informed no option is risk-free. Using ARR, provided it is the appropriate measure, may help reduce bias since the use of RRR tends to make changes in risk to appear larger.

In the chapter, we have provided an overview of the main issues of translation of evidence into practice. This is a significant challenge for evidence-based healthcare. In the next chapter, we will discuss how to also address under-representation in healthcare research before describing teaching and learning strategies for addressing some of these issues.

Understanding the risks of breast cancer

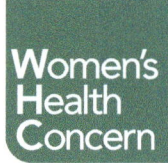

Women's Health Concern

A comparison of lifestyle risk factors versus hormone replacement therapy (HRT) treatment.

Difference in breast cancer incidence per 1000 women aged 50–59.
Approximate number of women developing breast cancer over the next five years.

NICE Guideline, Menopause: Diagnosis and management November 2015

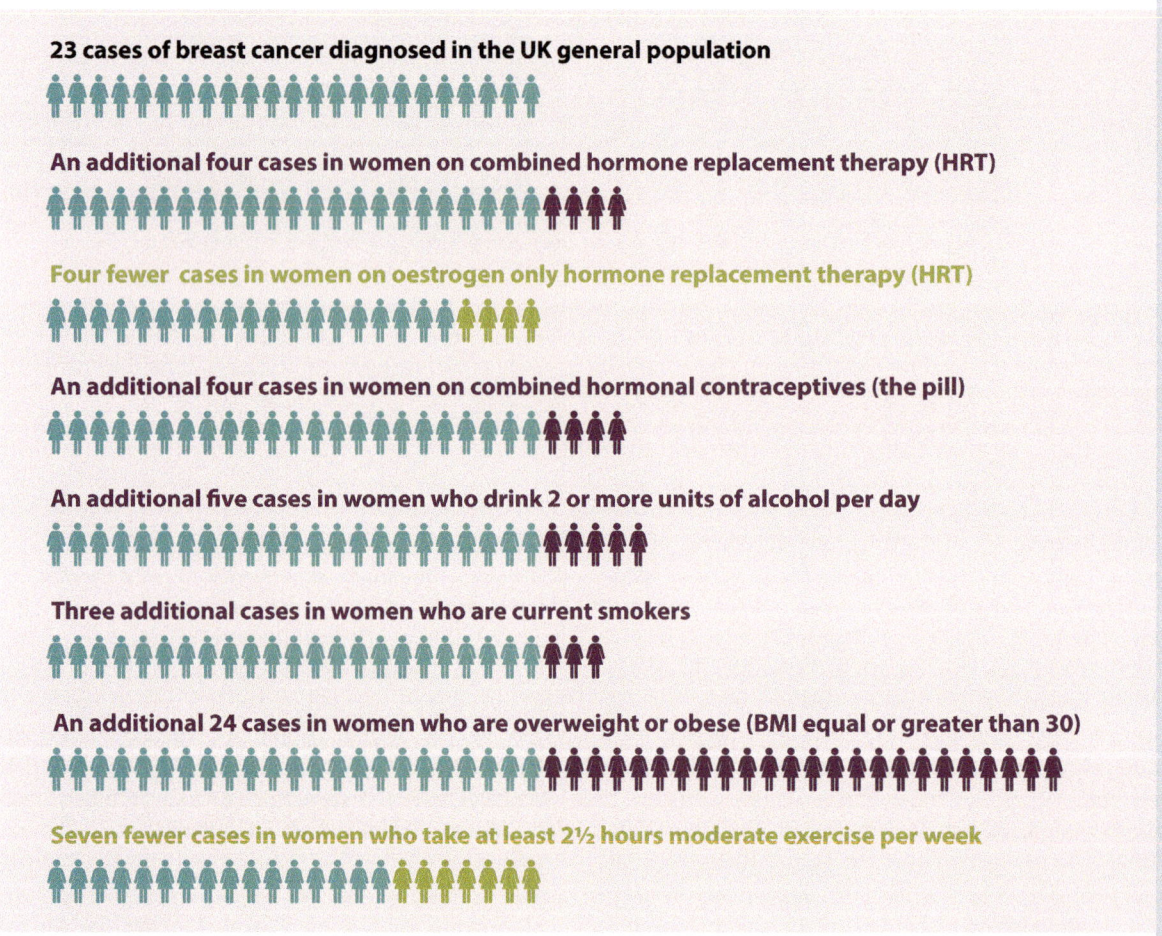

23 cases of breast cancer diagnosed in the UK general population

An additional four cases in women on combined hormone replacement therapy (HRT)

Four fewer cases in women on oestrogen only hormone replacement therapy (HRT)

An additional four cases in women on combined hormonal contraceptives (the pill)

An additional five cases in women who drink 2 or more units of alcohol per day

Three additional cases in women who are current smokers

An additional 24 cases in women who are overweight or obese (BMI equal or greater than 30)

Seven fewer cases in women who take at least 2½ hours moderate exercise per week

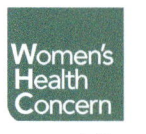

Women's Health Concern

www.womens-health-concern.org
Reg Charity No: 279651
Company Reg No: 1432023

Women's Health Concern is the patient arm of the BMS.
We provide an independent service to advise, reassure and educate women of all ages about their health, wellbeing and lifestyle concerns.

Go to **www.womens-health-concern.org**

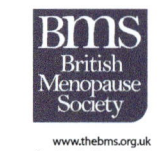

BMS
British Menopause Society

March 2017

www.thebms.org.uk
Reg Charity No: 1015144
Company Reg No: 02759439

Figure 8.9 PDA visualising the risks of breast cancer. *Source:* ABC of Clinical Reasoning, 2023/John Wiley & Sons.

Table 8.1 Measures of magnitude or effect size encountered in preventive screening.

Measure	Abbreviation	Calculation	Advantages and disadvantages in patient risk communication	Example (reduction in lung cancer mortality)
Natural frequency	NF	Number of persons with events in a population	• Highest levels of patient understanding and satisfaction • Denominator of 1000 people increases patient understanding of harms and benefits • Understanding increased when baseline risk is increased	13 of 1000 people died from lung cancer with screening; 16 of 1000 people died from lung cancer without screening. Thus, there were 3 of 1000 fewer deaths from lung cancer with screening
Absolute risk	AR	The number of events in the screened or control groups divided by the number of people in that group	• Increases patient understanding of risk • Understanding increased when baseline risk is included	AR in control group = 1.66% AR in screened group = 1.33%
Absolute risk reduction	ARR	Difference in the event rates between the screened and control arms of the study		ARR = 1.66%−1.33% = 0.33%
Relative risk	RR	Ratio of the outcome measure (e.g. mortality) in the screened group compared with the unscreened group	• Can cause exaggerated, perceived screening or treatment effects	RR = 0.80
Relative risk reduction	RRR	The difference in event rates between the screened and control groups divided by the event rate in the control group	• Can exaggerate the perceived treatment effect for both physicians and patients. Often presented as percentage without baseline risk	RRR = 1.66−1.33/1.66 = 0.20 RRR = 20%
Number needed to screen	NNS	Reciprocal of the ARR	• Decreased level of patient understanding compared with other measures of magnitude and effect size	NNS = 308[a]

All measures describe the same reduction in lung cancer mortality.
[a] Differs slightly from 1/ARR in this example due to rounding.
Source: Adapted from Bell et al. (19).

Box 8.3 **Discussion and record-keeping of shared decision-making of prescription of a statin in the primary prevention of cardiovascular disease**

Mrs Johal, 51 years, type 2 diabetes, obesity (BMI 34.4), no alcohol, never smoked. Normal blood pressure. Strong family history of stroke – Mum and uncle aged under 60 years. Seen to discuss results of cholesterol blood test. QRISK 3 20%

Discussed: Current UK guidelines – statin is advised if risk is >10%. Age and family history cannot be changed.
Risk increased due to type 2 diabetes. Reduce BMI, increase exercise and improve diet (lifestyle) to reduce risk.
Mrs Johal does not like taking tablets and knows family who take them. Wants to know the risks and benefits of taking/not taking statins.

We looked at NICE decision aid CG181 patient decision aid on whether should I take a statin (nice.org.uk).
Risk of a cardiac event (stroke or myocardial infarction) in the next 10 years is 20%. Out of 100 people with the same risk, 20 will get a cardiac event in the next 10 years. If she takes a statin, 7 would be prevented from getting the cardiac event – 13 would still get them.
Risks of muscle problems with statins are very low. Out of 100 people on a statin, 26 would get muscle pain anyway and 2 would get muscle pain due to the statin.

Plan
1 Link sent to decision aid.
2 Discuss with family.
3 Look at the lifestyle changes we discussed – wants to get BMI down to 25.
4 Review and reconsider with repeat cholesterol in three months.

Box 8.4 **Methods of communication of risk of a screening test where the benefits are equal for RRR, ARR and NNT**

• RRR – If you have this test every 2 years, it will reduce your chance of dying from this cancer by about one-third over the next 10 years.
• ARR – If you have this test, it will reduce your chance of dying from this cancer from around 3 in a 1000 to around 2 in a 1000 over the next 10 years.
• NNT – If around 1000 people have this test every 2 years, 1 person will be saved from dying from this cancer every 10 years.

Source: Adapted from Gigerenzer et al. (25).

References

1 Straus, S.E. and Holroyd-Leduc, J. (2008). Knowledge-to-action cycle. *Evid Based Med* 13 (4): 98–100. https://doi.org/10.1136/ebm.13.4.98-a. PMID: 18667658.

2 Balas, E.A. and Boren, S.A. (2000). Managing clinical knowledge for health care improvement. *Yearb Med Inform* 1: 65–70. PMID: 27699347.

3 Powell, B.J., Fernandez, M.E., Williams, N.J. et al. (2019). Enhancing the impact of implementation strategies in healthcare: a research agenda. *Front Public Health* 22 (7): 3. https://doi.org/10.3389/fpubh.2019.00003. PMID: 30723713; PMCID: PMC6350272.

4 Greenhalgh, T. and Papoutsi, C. (2019). Spreading and scaling up innovation and improvement. *BMJ* 10 (365): l2068. https://doi.org/10.1136/bmj.l2068. PMID: 31076440; PMCID: PMC6519511.

5 Horton, T.J., Illingworth, J.H., and Warburton, W.H.P. (2018). Overcoming challenges in codifying and replicating complex health care interventions. *Health Aff (Millwood)* 37 (2): 191–197. https://doi.org/10.1377/hlthaff.2017.1161. PMID: 29401020.

6 Dissemination & Implementation Models in Health Research and Practice (2019). https://dissemination-implementation.org/tool/ (accessed 24 August 2024).

7 Westgard, C. and Fleming, W.O. (2020). The use of implementation science tools to design, implement, and monitor a community-based mhealth intervention for child health in the amazon. *Front Public Health* 8: 411. https://doi.org/10.3389/fpubh.2020.00411.

8 Borsky, A., Zhan, C., Miller, T. et al. (2018). Few Americans receive all high-priority, appropriate clinical preventive services. *Health Aff (Millwood)* 37 (6): 925–928. https://doi.org/10.1377/hlthaff.2017.1248. PMID: 29863918.

9 Cooper, N., Bartlett, M., Gay, S. et al. (2021). UK clinical reasoning in medical education (CReME) consensus statement group. Consensus statement on the content of clinical reasoning curricula in undergraduate medical education. *Med Teach* 43 (2): 152–159. https://doi.org/10.1080/0142159X.2020.1842343. Epub 2020 Nov 18. PMID: 33205693.

10 Cooper, N. and Frain, J. (2023). *ABC of Clinical Reasoning*, 2e. Oxford: Wiley.

11 Silverman, J. (2017). *Chapter 2: The Consultation in ABC of Clinical Communication*. Oxford: Wiley.

12 Elwyn, G., Laitner, S., Coulter, A. et al. (2010). Implementing shared decision making in the NHS. *BMJ* 14 (341): c5146. https://doi.org/10.1136/bmj.c5146. PMID: 20947577.

13 Elwyn, G., Durand, M.A., Song, J. et al. (2017). A three-talk model for shared decision making: multistage consultation process. *BMJ* 6 (359): j4891. https://doi.org/10.1136/bmj.j4891. PMID: 29109079; PMCID: PMC5683042.

14 Morgan, D.J., Scherer, L.D., and Korenstein, D. (2020). Improving physician communication about treatment decisions: reconsideration of "risks vs benefits". *JAMA* 324 (10): 937–938. https://doi.org/10.1001/jama.2020.0354. PMID: 32150219.

15 Hoffmann, T.C., Légaré, F., Simmons, M.B. et al. (2014). Shared decision making: what do clinicians need to know and why should they bother? *Med J Aust* 201 (1): 35–39. https://doi.org/10.5694/mja14.00002. PMID: 24999896.

16 Barratt, A. (2008). Evidence based medicine and shared decision making: the challenge of getting both evidence and preferences into health care. *Patient Educ Couns* 73 (3): 407–412. https://doi.org/10.1016/j.pec.2008.07.054. Epub 2008 Oct 8. PMID: 18845414.

17 Stacey, D., Lewis, K.B., Smith, M. et al. (2024). Decision aids for people facing health treatment or screening decisions. *Cochrane Database Syst Rev 1* (1): CD001431. https://doi.org/10.1002/14651858.CD001431.pub6. PMID: 38284415; PMCID: PMC10823577.

18 Baccolini, V., Rosso, A., Di Paolo, C. et al. (2021). What is the prevalence of low health literacy in European union member states? A systematic review and meta-analysis. *J Gen Intern Med* 36 (3): 753–761. https://doi.org/10.1007/s11606-020-06407-8. Epub 2021 Jan 5. PMID: 33403622; PMCID: PMC7947142.

19 Bell, N.R., Dickinson, J.A., Grad, R. et al. (2018). Understanding and communicating risk: measures of outcome and the magnitude of benefits and harms. *Can Fam Physician* 64 (3): 181–185. PMID: 29540382; PMCID: PMC5851390.

20 Richter, R., Jansen, J., Bongaerts, I. et al. (2023). Communication of benefits and harms in shared decision making with patients with limited health literacy: a systematic review of risk communication strategies. *Patient Educ Couns* 116: 107944. https://doi.org/10.1016/j.pec.2023.107944. Epub 2023 Aug 17. PMID: 37619376.

21 Stacey, D., Légaré, F., Lewis, K. et al. (2017). Decision aids for people facing health treatment or screening decisions. *Cochrane Database Syst Rev* 4 (4): CD001431. doi: https://doi.org/10.1002/14651858.CD001431.pub5.

22 Noseworthy, P.A., Brito, J.P., Kunneman, M. et al. (2019). Shared decision-making in atrial fibrillation: navigating complex issues in partnership with the patient. *J Interv Card Electrophysiol* 56 (2): 159–163. https://doi.org/10.1007/s10840-018-0465-5. Epub 2018 Oct 17. PMID: 30327992; PMCID: PMC7056296.

23 Elwyn, G., Lloyd, A., Joseph-Williams, N. et al. (2013). Option grids: shared decision making made easier. *Patient Educ Couns* 90 (2): 207–212. https://doi.org/10.1016/j.pec.2012.06.036. Epub 2012 Jul 31. PMID: 22854227.

24 Johnston, B.C., Alonso-Coello, P., Friedrich, J.O. et al. (2016). Do clinicians understand the size of treatment effects? A randomized survey across 8 countries. *CMAJ* 188 (1): 25–32. https://doi.org/10.1503/cmaj.150430. Epub 2015 Oct 26. PMID: 26504102; PMCID: PMC4695351.

25 Gigerenzer, G., Gaissmaier, W., Kurz-Milcke, E. et al. (2007). Helping doctors and patients make sense of health statistics. *Psychol Sci Public Interest* 8 (2): 53–96. https://doi.org/10.1111/j.1539-6053.2008.00033.x. Epub 2007 Nov 1. PMID: 26161749.

26 Edwards, A. and Trevana, L. (2016). What you need to know as a clinician about risk communication, chapter 18. In: *Shared Decision Making in Health Care: Achieving Evidence-based Patient Choice*, 3e (ed. G. Elwyn), 112–122. Oxford: Oxford University Press.

Further reading

Elwyn, G. (2016). *Shared Decision Making in Health Care: Achieving Evidence-based Patient Choice*, 3e. Oxford: Oxford University Press.

Greenhalgh, T. (2017). *How to Implement Evidence-based Healthcare*. Oxford: Wiley-Blackwell.

Hammond, A. and Gay, S. (2023). *Shared Decision Making, Chapter in ABC of Clinical Decision Making, Chapter in ABC of Clinical Reasoning*, 2e. Oxford: Wiley.

Sackett, D.L., Rosenberg, W.M., Gray, J.A. et al. (1996) Evidence based medicine: what it is and what it isn't. BMJ 312(7023): 71–72.

Wearn, A. and Frain, J. (2017). *Shared Decision Making, chapter in ABC of Clinical Communication*. Oxford: Wiley.

CHAPTER 9

Challenges in Evidence-Based Healthcare

John Frain

Division of Medical Sciences and Graduate Entry Medicine, University of Nottingham, Nottingham, UK

OVERVIEW

- Representation and inclusion in healthcare research needs to improve for outcomes to be applicable to all patients.
- Principles of inclusion should be incorporated into study design throughout the cycle.
- Artificial intelligence (AI) may improve the quality and amount of information available to clinicians.
- The application of AI to automation of guidelines, evidence summaries and evidence quality is increasing rapidly, though knowledge gaps may exist currently in the finished articles.
- Evidence-based healthcare has challenges for the future rather than limitations, though these are not insurmountable.

Inclusion in research

In a study of clinical trials across 29 countries between 1997 and 2014, 86% of subjects were identified as White (1). In the United Kingdom, White British people are 64% more likely than ethnic minorities to have participated in clinical research even when accounting for socioeconomic status, age and gender (2). Consequently, populations at particular risk of a condition may not be included in the studies designed to understand the disease and test new treatments (3). For example, while Black patients were 54% more likely to develop dementia over a 10-year period, a review of 83 clinical trials of drugs for Alzheimer's disease found only 2% of subjects were Black (3). These statistics are reflected more generally in healthcare, where there are differing rates of access to hospital services between groups of different ethnicities. For example, Hispanic patients are less likely to be referred to outpatient neurology than Whites, while Blacks are more likely to present with neurological conditions as emergency patients (4). There was under-representation of ethnic minorities in Covid-19 trials for treatments, immunisation and other research. This is despite the greater incidence of Covid-19 in these groups. Evidence-based healthcare may routinely forget the needs and perspectives of marginalised groups. Patients from ethnic minorities have been consistently found to receive poorer care than White patients in many illnesses. Contributing to this is a lack of research in their populations as well as bias towards them.

Similarly, the LGBTQIA+ community is generally disregarded in trial design or research done may be skewed. For example, nearly three-quarters of published studies on neurological conditions in LGBTQIA+ patients focus on HIV-positive individuals, making the results non-generalisable to non-HIV patients (5). Approaches to patient selection which select solely on the basis of gender assigned at birth may overlook patient groups with factors associated with particular risks, for example, of mental health and well-being conditions. Representation in research is lacking in minority ethnic populations, older adults, women, pregnant and breastfeeding individuals, LGBTQIA+ people, migrants, sex workers, homeless and persons with disabilities (Box 9.1) (3).

Historical abuses as well as personal experiences can affect confidence in accessing services. Following revelation of the Tuskegee syphilis study in Alabama (Box 9.2), Black men were less likely to trust doctors, reduced contact with services and suffered increased mortality (6). Persisting lack of diversity in clinical trials facilitates the perception that healthcare is not inclusive of everyone. The importance of this is illustrated by a study where patients were randomly given the results of two trials of a new drug for hypertension. Both showed the new drug treated hypertension effectively. In one trial, less than 1% of participants were Black; in the other, 15% of participants were Black. The results of the more representative trial increased the belief among Black patients that the drug would be effective for them without altering the perceptions of the White patients (7).

Trial sponsors have advocated equity, diversity and inclusion (EDI) to be incorporated into the complete cycle of clinical trials (Figure 9.1) (3). Stakeholders, including patients and their families, should be involved in trial design. The protocol should address difficulties around participation, such as the ease of visiting the research centre. There may be justification for remote participation online, dependent on trial requirements. The language of patient information for recruitment should be inclusive and address health literacy needs in the target population. Intention to treat analyses should ensure participants are not lost to follow-up due to engagement issues, financial difficulties or bias. Barriers to engagement in research include patient vulnerability, perceived risk of participation, mistrust of medical research and participant resources (e.g. travel and childcare).

Box 9.1 Sex differences in symptom presentation in acute coronary syndrome (ACS)

ACS and angina may present differently in men and women. Women can have different symptoms compared to men, but there is also a substantial overlap. Chest pain is the most common symptom in both sexes. In a systematic review published in 2020, women had higher odds of pain between scapulae, nausea or vomiting and shortness of breath. Women have lower odds of chest pain and diaphoresis.

These differences have been known about for over 20 years but are not yet in mainstream clinical practice, meaning women are late to being diagnosed, late to treatment and with a consequent impact on prognosis. In 2021, the American Heart Association published its first guideline on chest pain in women, stating, 'In women presenting with chest pain, it is recommended to obtain a history that emphasises accompanying symptoms that are more common in women with ACS' (26).

Source: Adapted from van Oosterhout et al. (27).

Box 9.2 The Tuskegee Untreated Syphilis Study, Alabama, US

In 1932, the US Public Health Service (USPHS) began a study to record the natural history of syphilis, a sexually transmitted disease. The study followed 600 Black men, 399 of whom had syphilis and 201 without the disease. Participants were told they were being treated for 'bad blood'. Informed consent about the true purpose of the study was not obtained. In return for taking part in the study, the men were provided with free medical examination, free meals and burial insurance. During the study, 28 men (and possibly up to 100) died of the direct effects of syphilis, while another 154 died of heart failure. It is not known how many patients' deaths were connected to syphilis.

In 1943, penicillin became widely available and was the treatment of choice for syphilis. Participants in the study were not offered treatment. The study did not become public until a leaked story appeared in the Associated Press in 1972. An advisory panel advised the study was 'ethically unjustified' and it was discontinued shortly thereafter. It was not until 1997 that President Clinton issued a formal presidential apology.

Source: Adaptef from Centers for Disease Control and Prevention (28).

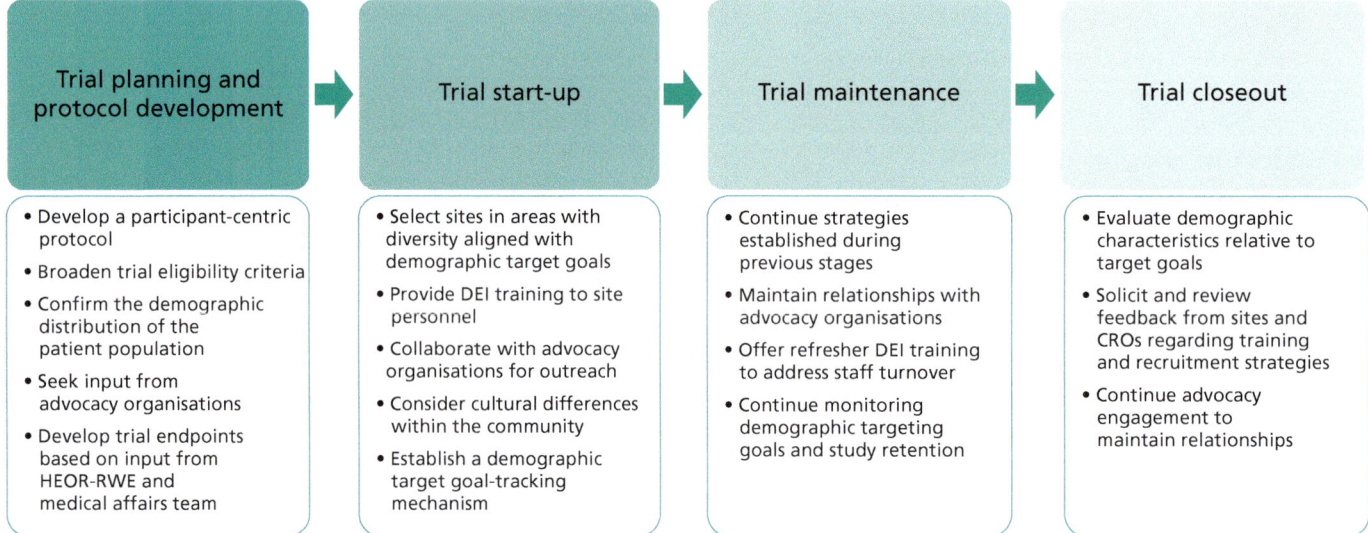

Figure 9.1 Tool for diversity, equity and inclusion within the clinical trial lifecycle. CRO, contract research organisation; HEOR-RWE, health economics outcomes research and real-world evidence. *Source:* Versavel et al. (3)/with permission of Elsevier.

Sampling issues may affect the external validity of research. Underpowered studies may not contain large enough subgroups to permit sufficient statistical analysis. A review in 2011 of 86 trials found only 25% reported gender-specific results, while 64% did not report an analysis of groups by ethnicity (8). Toolkits exist to help address equality in UK research (9). Ethnicity and other protected characteristics should be recorded, where relevant to outcomes, at the outset of a study and then on publication of the report. This should be reflected in research regulations. Figure 9.2 shows a model for health research inclusivity (10).

Artificial intelligence

The evidence base of healthcare increases exponentially. It exceeds the capacity of any one individual to comprehend it (Box 9.3). The time lag between generation of evidence and effective implementation in practice can be as long as 17 years (11). AI and machine learning (ML) are proposed as technologies to automate the retrieval and analysis of biomedical literature (12). AI is computer-based algorithms simulating human intelligence. Their use allows computers to perform tasks previously requiring human

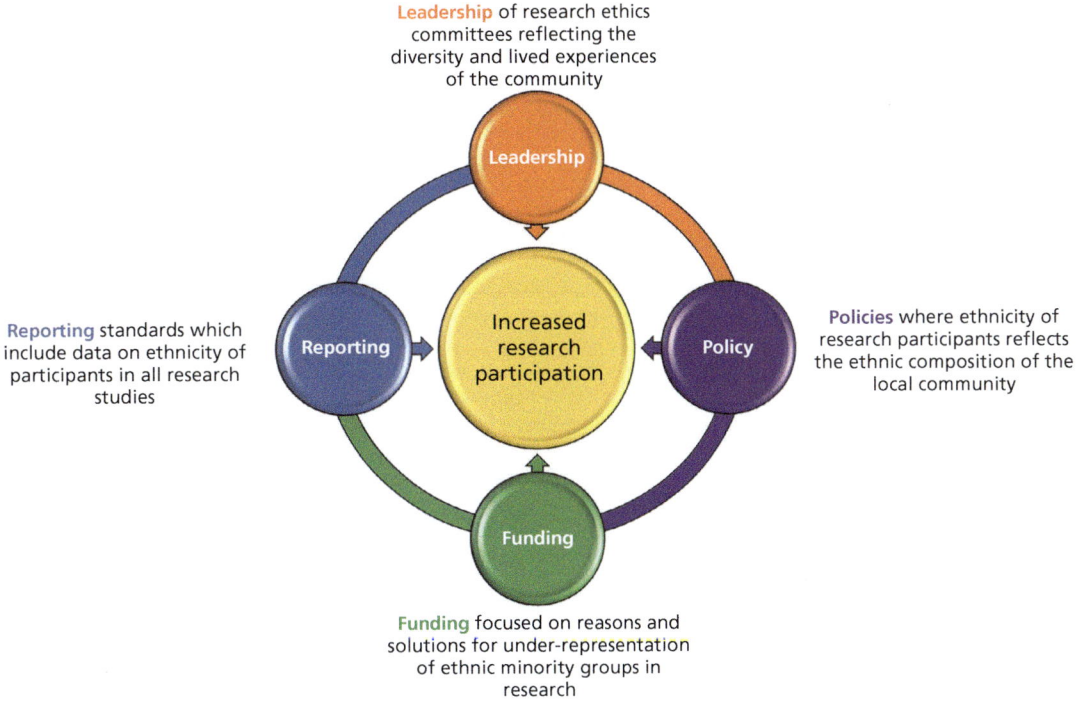

Figure 9.2 Health research inclusivity model. *Source:* Osuafor et al. (10)/with permission of Elsevier.

At medical school we were told half of what we were taught would be wrong in 10 years – no one knew which half. Certain facts were drilled in as being so definite that years later it could be hard to change practice.

1. Having been taught never to prescribe beta blockers in heart failure, it is counter-intuitive when the guidelines change. It can be hard to override the ingrained advice.
2. After years of prescribing warfarin, replacing it with an non-vitamin K oral anticoagulants (NOAC) can feel challenging.
3. New advice that MRI scans of the prostate replace rectal examinations means as a GP, rectal examinations are not essential before a referral. However, I might feel I am not doing a thorough job if I do not do this.
4. Urine in the over 65 age group should not be dipped. This has been known for many years and yet in care homes, GP surgeries and hospital dipping still happens.

Why does new evidence take so long to be taken up by clinicians on the ground? What can I do to improve?

Recognising my own inertia. Keeping up with new guidelines. Learning about the side effects and risks of new medication. Listening to colleagues, learning together and sharing knowledge. Improving my shared decision-making skills and communicating risk to patients.

Good understanding by EBM leaders and researchers of the challenges facing frontline clinicians could help to develop ways of embedding new knowledge into practice.

Reflection: Dr Anna Frain

cognitive skills (12). AI is rapidly developing its own terminology (Box 9.4). The literature of AI in medicine has increased dramatically in recent years (Figure 9.3).

A scoping review of the evidence identified three main uses of AI in evidence-based healthcare thus far: Group I – the assembly of scientific evidence, Group II – mining the biomedical literature and Group III – quality analysis (12). AI is now used in screening, identification and selection of studies for systematic reviews. The first reported use was in 2006 with a marked increase after 2018. Elements of PICO question construction can be extracted using the algorithms defined in Box 9.4. Reporting, critical appraisal and risk of bias tools were used to assess quality. A systematic review of the use of AI in evidence synthesis reported that although the number of published studies is rapidly increasing, it is currently difficult to draw firm conclusions about the accuracy of AI in this context due to the heterogeneity of the published evidence (13). Knowledge gaps exist in automated construction of guidelines, preparation of evidence summaries and analysis of quality. This means further development is required for them to be safely used in practice.

At the same time, there has been rapid progress in quality in evidence synthesis in areas such as diabetic retinopathy, glaucoma and chest imaging. This was also evident during Covid-19, when rapid reviews facilitated the implementation of management strategies to reduce morbidity and mortality (14). Clinical trials are complex processes which are both labour- and data-intensive (Figure 9.4). AI's ability to analyse rapidly vast amounts of data is valuable at all stages of development. This includes identification of potential recruits from, for example, electronic

Box 9.4 **Abbreviations and definitions in AI**

Abbreviation	Meaning	Definition
AI	Artificial intelligence	Computer-based algorithms simulating human intelligence
DL	Deep learning	A subset of machine learning which uses deep neural networks to simulate the complex decision-making of the human brain
IoMT	Internet of medical things	Inter-networked devices and applications used in medical and healthcare information technology
KNN	k-Nearest neighbours	A non-parametric learning classifier which uses proximity of other data to classify or make predictions about an individual data point. Popular and simple classifier used in machine learning
LLM	Large language model	A computer model capable of language generation or natural language processing tasks
ML	Machine learning	An application enabling computers to learn from their mistakes and predict results without explicit programming to do so
MLP	Multilayer perceptron	An artificial neural network comprised of multiple layers of neurons
MLR	Multinomial logistic regression	The outcome variable is nominal and has more than two categories that do not have a given rank or order
NER	Named entity recognition	A component of natural language processing that identifies predefined categories in a text
NLL	Natural processing language	A component of deep learning which enables computers to understand and analyse human language – used in the interpretation of electronic medical records and scientific articles
RWD	Real-world data	Data that come from sources other than clinical trials
SGD	Stochastic gradient descent	An optimisation algorithm used in machine learning to find model parameters which best fit between predicted and actual outputs
SVM	Support vector machine	A supervised machine learning algorithm which classifies data through finding an optimal line to maximise the distance between each class

Source: Adapted from Santos et al. (12)/with permission of Elsevier.

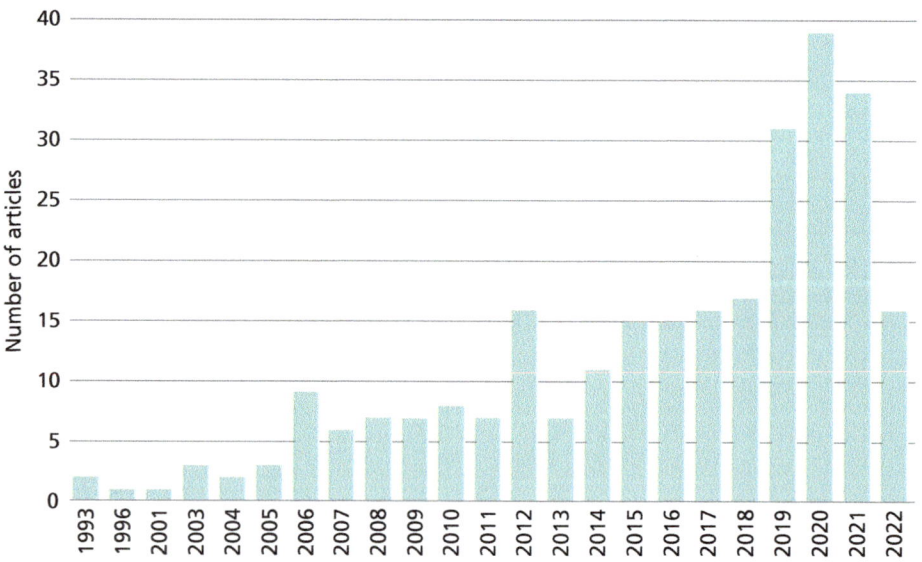

Figure 9.3 Number of articles on the use of AI for automating or semi-automating biomedical literature analyses and year of publication. *Source:* Santos et al. (12)/with permission of Elsevier.

patient records and social media (Figure 9.5) (15). In-depth data analysis facilitates clinician's understanding of population patterns and patient needs. Increased data capture and analysis may facilitate prediction of clinical outcomes and prognosis. Conversely, there are concerns around privacy, data protection and patient consent. Algorithms will extract predefined datasets which will lead to homogenised sampling in patient recruitment. The algorithms on which AI are trained will, at least in the

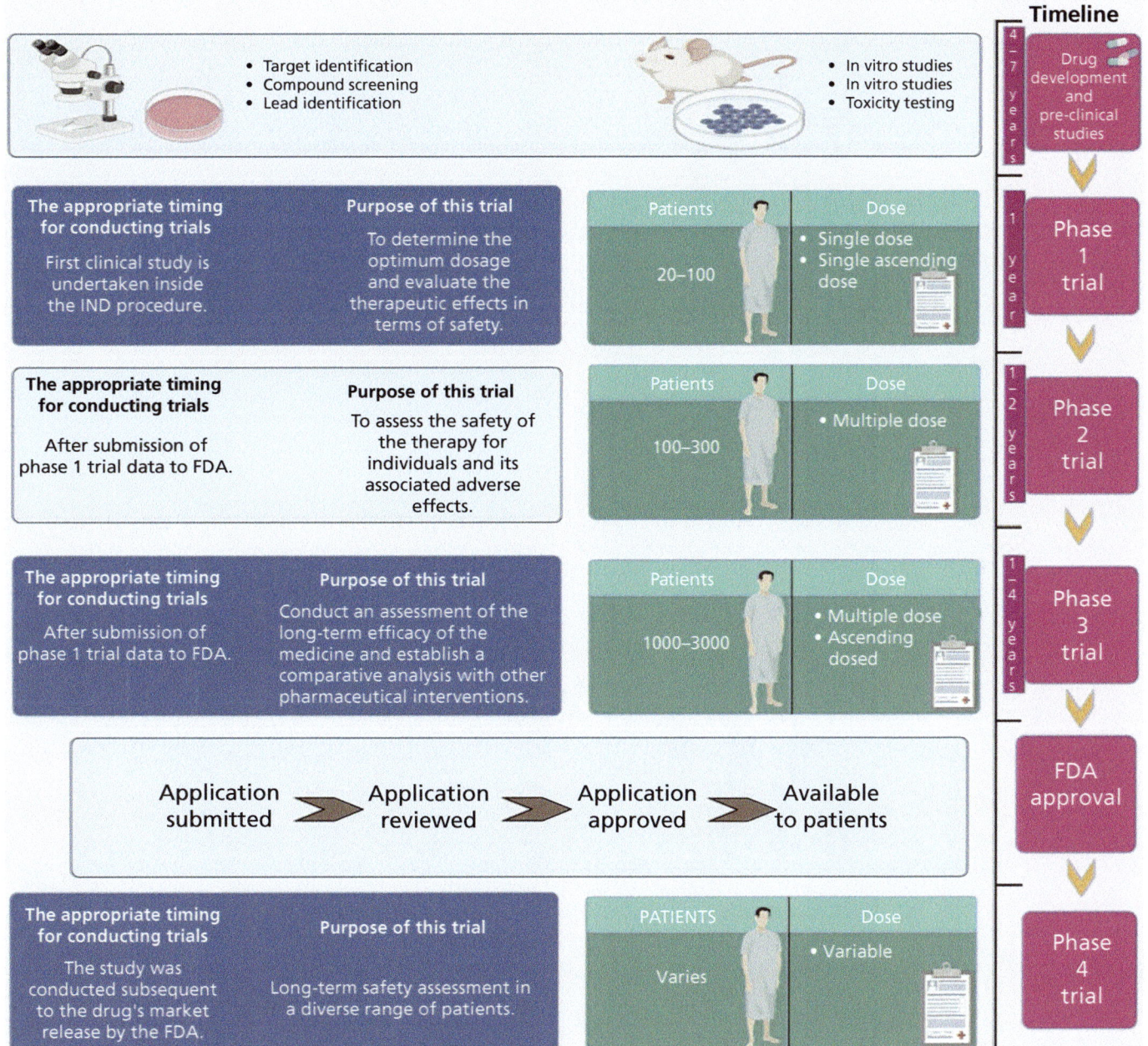

Figure 9.4 Steps in US Food and Drug Administration drug approval for clinical trials. *Source:* Chopra et al. (15)/JMIR Publications/CC BY 4.0.

short term, continue to contain the bias towards Caucasian and women populations already prevalent in research studies. This is yet another imperative for improving representation and inclusion in research (15). This is being addressed through amended reporting guidelines such as SPIRIT-AI and CONSORT-AI (16, 17). Currently, patient safety assessments of AI-enabled healthcare research are limited in number, with only one study reporting it as a major outcome (18).

'Listen to the patient and their data; they are telling you the diagnosis'

We are on the frontier of an explosion in the availability to front-line clinicians of patient's clinical and biomedical data. While we will, with greater understanding than ever before, still listen to the patient's history and examine for physical evidence of established disease in the patient's body and mind, we will also have

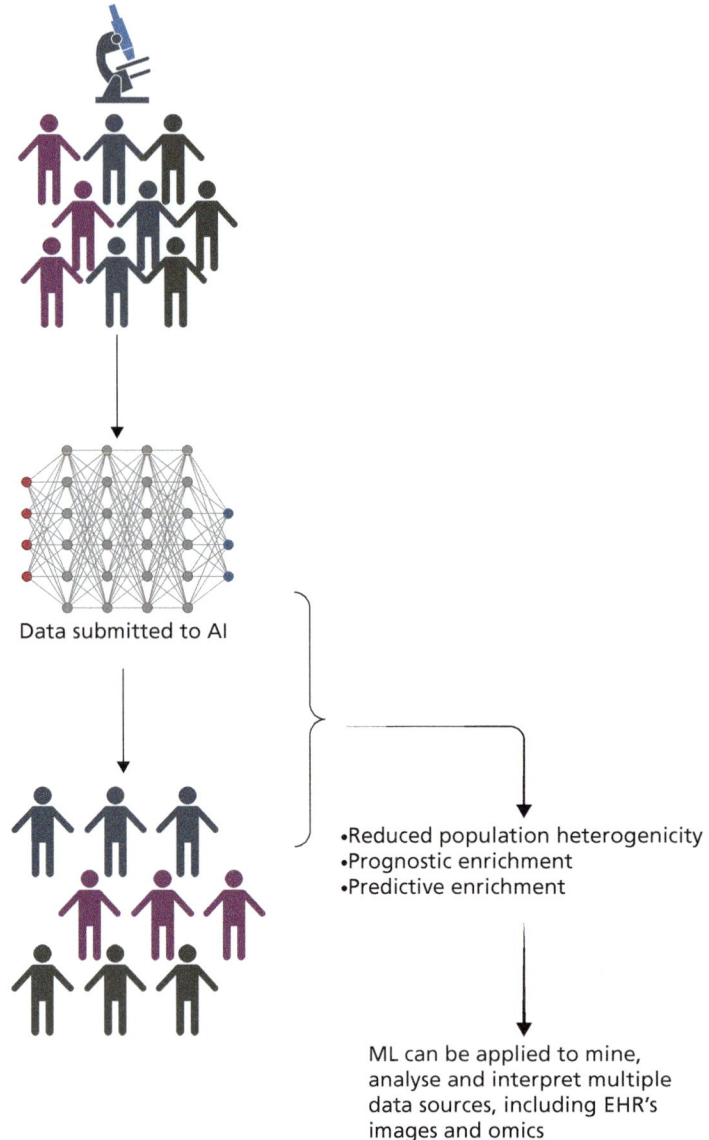

Data submitted to AI

•Reduced population heterogenicity
•Prognostic enrichment
•Predictive enrichment

ML can be applied to mine,
analyse and interpret multiple
data sources, including EHR's
images and omics

Figure 9.5 Use of AI in clinical trials. *Source:* Chopra et al. (15)/JMIR Publications/CC BY 4.0.

available synthesised evidence from populations and the individual patient in our personal evidence micro-cart. Our existing evidence pyramids, however they are modelled, have been described as the tip of an iceberg merely suggestive of the mass of data lying beneath which will enable us to personalise patient's medical care to their particular needs, preferences and values (Figure 9.6) (19).

Are there limitations to evidence-based healthcare?

This book summarises the achievements of evidence-based healthcare and outlines areas for further development. Clinicians of the twenty-first century are more greatly aware of the benefits of systematic evidence review and its benefits for patient care. Guidelines provide more structured patient care and improve patient outcomes.

Evidence-based healthcare has improved objectivity in clinical decision-making. Criticism does arise from an over-concentration in research on treatments and devices (20). It has taken longer to take account, through qualitative research, of the perspective of both patient and clinician in implementing patient care. Safe clinical practice also requires evidence of appropriate health policies, service management and delivery. Mechanistic reasoning and clinical judgement both remain important in the application of population-based studies to the individual patient (20). Building confidence among the frontline clinicians who must apply the evidence is crucial, and any perceived shortcoming in the selection of evidence for review risks undermining evidence-based healthcare (21). Notions and models of evidence hierarchies have assisted clinicians in how to understand and approach the critical appraisal of evidence. The achievements and limitations of evidence-based healthcare are summarised in Table 9.1 (20).

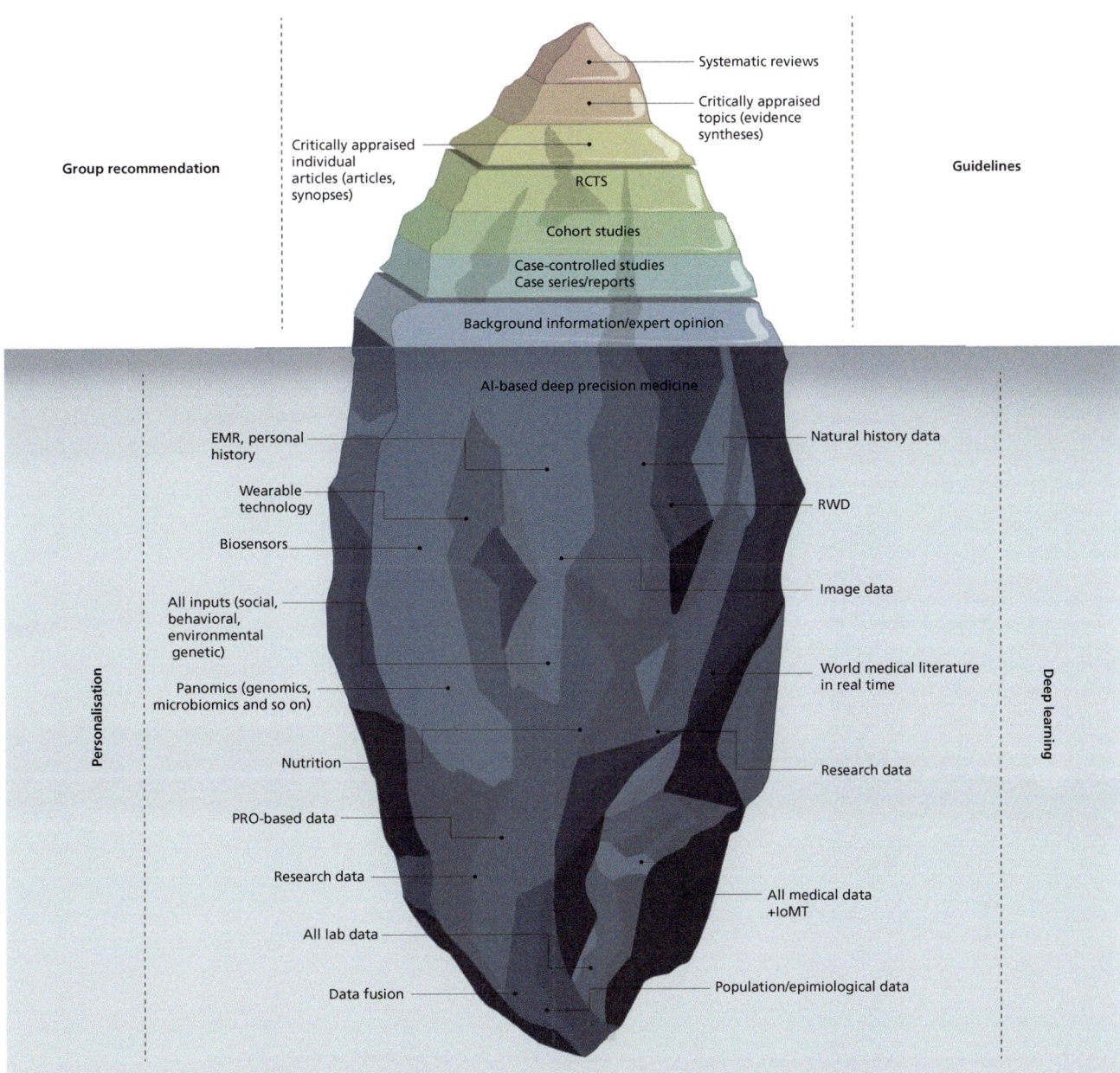

The current evidence-based medicine (EBM) pyramid represents the tip of the iceberg and barely provides enough shallow evidence to care for a generic patient. Hence, a deep synthesis and amalgamation of all available data is needed to achieve next-generation, deep evidence-based medicine. The main challenge ahead in the next two decades will be extracting, collating and mining large sets of natural history data, genomics and all omics analyses, all published clinical studies, RWD and amassed data from the IoMT to provide next-generation evidence for deep medicine. PRO, patient-reported outcomes.

Figure 9.6 Evidence-based deep medicine iceberg. *Source:* Subbiah (19)/with permission of Springer Nature.

An early criticism of evidence-based healthcare was that it represented 'cookbook medicine' and discounted the experience and judgement of individual clinicians who must take ultimate responsibility for patient care (22). While emphasising objective evidence, evidence-based healthcare can be perceived as failing to take account of the complexity and intangible factors occurring in patient care (23). The relationship between evidence, clinical judgement and the individual patient has not always been clear, although 'evidence can never directly dictate care: the evidence cannot tell us when it is best to ignore the evidence' (23). These concerns are reflected in commentaries throughout the last 30-plus years (24). This is not to be disrespectful of the achievement of evidence-based healthcare. A healthy scepticism and a willingness to critically appraise the methodology are exactly the attitudes and skills the leaders of the evidence-based medicine (EBM) movement have sought to promote in healthcare. The emphasis on evidence, structure, systematic review and appraisal are tenets now allowing us to combine evidence-based healthcare with personalised medicine (Figure 9.7) (25).

Table 9.1 Achievements and limitations of EBM.

- Efforts to improve the evidence base of medicine have a long history over several centuries.
- The EBM movement – a group of epidemiologists from McMaster University launched EBM in the early 1990s.
  - Claimed to have initiated a 'new paradigm' of medical practice
  - Advocated greater reliance on published data in clinical practice
  - Proposed a hierarchy of evidence, with clinical trials trumping mechanistic reasoning
- The Cochrane collaboration – founded in the United Kingdom with Department of Health sponsorship by members of the EBM movement.
  - Expanded capacity to 40000 volunteers worldwide
  - Produces reviews of published research, mainly related to drugs and devices
  - Contributed to the development of clinical guidelines
  - Advocacy and campaigning – calls for full disclosure of clinical trials
  - Contributed to the awareness of 'overdiagnosis' and campaigns against 'too much medicine'
- Limitations of EBM – relegation of clinical judgement and mechanistic reasoning, and over-reliance on the reliability of clinical trials and systematic reviews.
- Limitation of clinical trials and systematic reviews due to:
  - Unrepresentativeness of trial patients in terms of age, therapy and comorbidity
  - Over-reliance on statistical as opposed to clinical significance
  - Misleading results due to reporting bias, inappropriate pooling of small trials, effect of changes in disease mortality and progress over time
- Adverse effects on clinical practice: bias of the 'easily measurable' risks relegating less tangible values, such as patient experience, dignity and knowledge creation.
  - Biases of commissioned research can reduce independence of topics selected for study and distort the evidence base.
  - An exclusive focus on drugs and devices has left large aspects of health in an evidence vacuum.
- Conflation of comparative research and original science: comparative research evaluates what is known, and original science seeks to explore what is unknown.
  - Expansion of comparative science since the launch of EBM contributed to a decline in original clinical science.
  - Over-reliance on comparative research distorts what is needed to meet some future challenges.
    - 'Overdiagnosis' is seen as a problem of 'too much medicine' leading to campaigns to 'do less', ignoring durable solutions that require novel approaches relying on new knowledge.
    - 'Antibiotic resistance' is too often presented as a problem of inappropriate use, ignoring the need to find new ways to combat infection.
- The future of EBM – relocated within the wider context of medicine and medical science:
  - The principle of medical professionalism is not limited to a process of drug and device evaluation
  - Independent of all interests, whether commercial, ideological or political
  - Allied to, but separate from, and serving a different function than original science

Source: Sheridan et al. (20)/with permission of Elsevier.

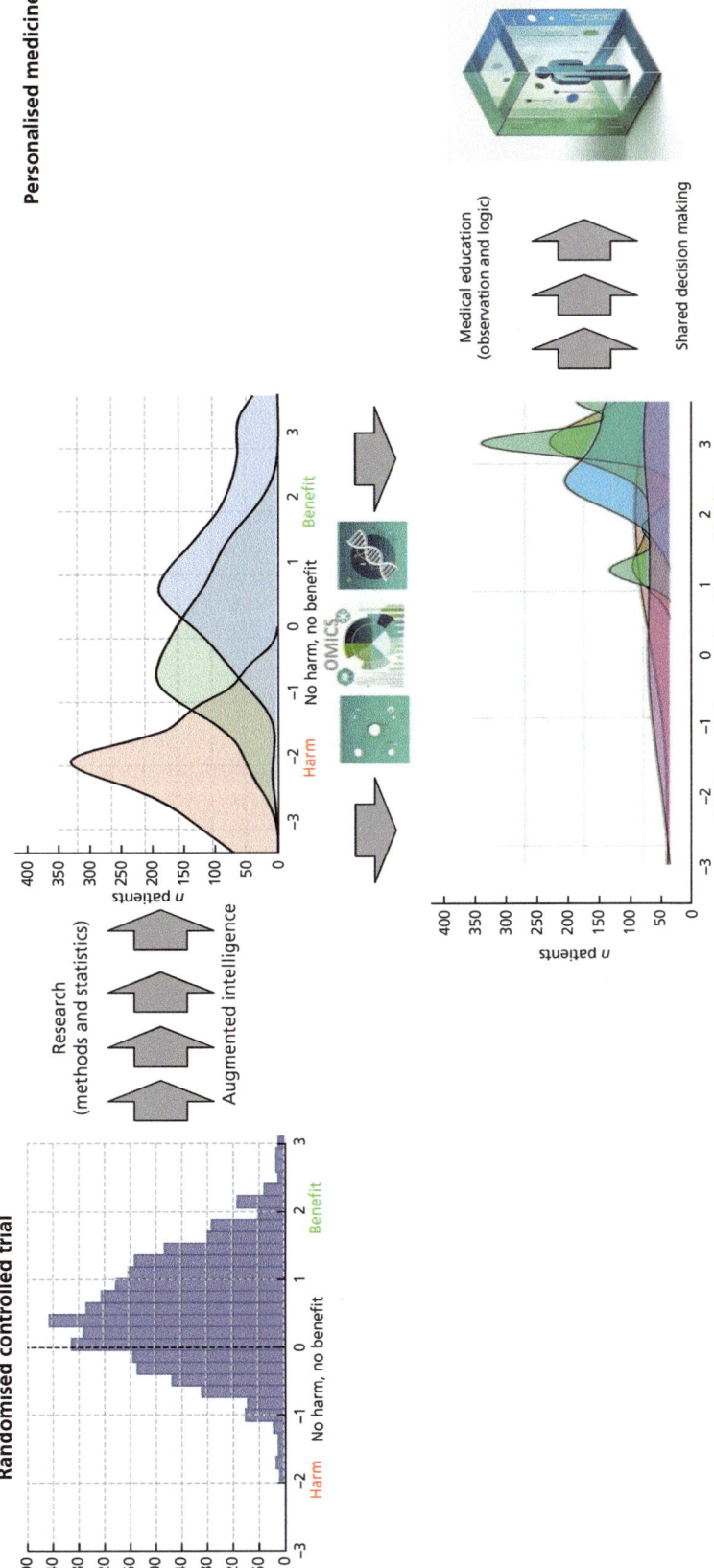

Figure 9.7 From randomised controlled trials to personalised medicine. *Source:* Adapted from Einav and O'Connor (25).

References

1 Knepper, T.C. and McLeod, H.L. (2018). When will clinical trials finally reflect diversity? *Nature* 557 (7704): 157–159.

2 Khunti, K., Bellary, S., Karamat, M.A. et al. (2017). Representation of people of South Asian origin in cardiovascular outcome trials of glucose-lowering therapies in Type 2 diabetes. *Diabet Med* 34 (1): 64–68.

3 Versavel, S., Subasinghe, A., Johnson, K. et al. (2023). Diversity, equity, and inclusion in clinical trials: a practical guide from the perspective of a trial sponsor. *Contemp Clin Trials* 126: 107092.

4 Saadi, A., Himmelstein, D.U., Woolhandler, S., and Mejia, N.I. (2017). Racial disparities in neurologic health care access and utilization in the United States. *Neurology* 88 (24): 2268–2275.

5 Rosendale, N., Wong, J.O., Flatt, J.D., and Whitaker, E. (2021). Sexual and gender minority health in neurology: a scoping review. *JAMA Neurol* 78 (6): 747–754.

6 Alsan, M. and Wanamaker, M. (2018). Tuskegee and the health of black men. *Q J Econ* 133 (1): 407–455.

7 Alsan, M., Durvasula, M., Gupta, H. et al. (2024). Representation and extrapolation: evidence from clinical trials. *Q J Econ* 139 (1): 575–635.

8 Geller, S.E., Koch, A., Pellettieri, B., and Carnes, M. (2011). Inclusion, analysis, and reporting of sex and race/ethnicity in clinical trials: have we made progress? *J Women's Health (Larchmt)* 20 (3): 315–320.

9 NIHR (2024). National institute for health and care research applied research collaboration east midlands. Equality impact assessment (EqIA) toolkit. https://arc-em.nihr.ac.uk/arc-store-resources/equality-impact-assessment-eqia-toolkit (accessed 20 November 2024).

10 Osuafor, C.N., Golubic, R., and Ray, S. (2021). Ethnic inclusivity and preventative health research in addressing health inequalities and developing evidence base. *EClinicalMedicine* 31: 100672.

11 Morris, Z.S., Wooding, S., and Grant, J. (2011). The answer is 17 years, what is the question: understanding time lags in translational research. *J R Soc Med* 104 (12): 510–520.

12 Santos, Á.O.D., da Silva, E.S., Couto, L.M. et al. (2023). The use of artificial intelligence for automating or semi-automating biomedical literature analyses: a scoping review. *J Biomed Inform* 142: 104389.

13 Feng, Y., Liang, S., Zhang, Y. et al. (2022). Automated medical literature screening using artificial intelligence: a systematic review and meta-analysis. *J Am Med Inform Assoc* 29 (8): 1425–1432.

14 Chang, Z., Zhan, Z., Zhao, Z. et al. (2021). Application of artificial intelligence in COVID-19 medical area: a systematic review. *J Thorac Dis* 13 (12): 7034–7053.

15 Chopra, H., Annu, S.D.K., Munjal, K. et al. (2023). Revolutionizing clinical trials: the role of AI in accelerating medical breakthroughs. *Int J Surg* 109 (12): 4211–4220.

16 Rivera, S.C., Liu, X., Chan, A.W. et al. (2020). Guidelines for clinical trial protocols for interventions involving artificial intelligence: the SPIRIT-AI Extension. *BMJ* 370: m3210.

17 Liu, X., Cruz Rivera, S., Moher, D. et al. (2020). Reporting guidelines for clinical trial reports for interventions involving artificial intelligence: the CONSORT-AI extension. *Lancet Digit Health* 2 (10): e537–e548.

18 Laranjo, L., Dunn, A.G., Tong, H.L. et al. (2018). Conversational agents in healthcare: a systematic review. *J Am Med Inform Assoc* 25 (9): 1248–1258.

19 Subbiah, V. (2023). The next generation of evidence-based medicine. *Nat Med* 29 (1): 49–58.

20 Sheridan, D.J. and Julian, D.G. (2016). Achievements and limitations of evidence-based medicine. *J Am Coll Cardiol* 68 (2): 204–213.

21 Chu, E.Y., Stein, J.A., and Ming, M.E. (2020). Evaluation of the merits and limitations of evidence-based medicine. *JAMA Dermatol* 156 (8): 924–925.

22 Hasnain-Wynia, R. (2006). Is evidence-based medicine patient-centered and is patient-centered care evidence-based? *Health Serv Res* 41 (1): 1–8.

23 Tonelli, M.R. (1998). The philosophical limits of evidence-based medicine. *Acad Med* 73 (12): 1234–1240.

24 Fernandez, A., Sturmberg, J., Lukersmith, S. et al. (2015). Evidence-based medicine: is it a bridge too far? *Health Res Policy Syst* 13: 66.

25 Einav, S. and O'Connor, M. (2024). The limitations of evidence-based medicine compel the practice of personalized medicine. *Intensive Care Med* 50 (8): 1323–1326.

26 Kaur, G., Oliveira-Gomes, D., Rivera, F.B., and Gulati, M. (2023). Chest pain in women: considerations from the 2021 AHA/ACC chest pain guideline. *Curr Probl Cardiol* 48 (7): 101697.

27 van Oosterhout, R.E.M., de Boer, A.R., Maas, A. et al. (2020). Sex differences in symptom presentation in acute coronary syndromes: a systematic review and meta-analysis. *J Am Heart Assoc* 9 (9): e014733.

28 Centers for Disease Control and Prevention (2024). The USPHS untreated syphilis study at tuskegee: center for communicable diseases. https://www.cdc.gov/tuskegee/about/index.html#:~:text=The%20U.S.%20Public%20Health%20Service%20(USPHS)%20Untreated%20Syphilis%20Study%20at,after%20it%20was%20widely%20available (accessed 20 November 2024).

CHAPTER 10

Teaching and Learning Evidence-Based Healthcare

John Frain

Division of Medical Sciences and Graduate Entry Medicine, University of Nottingham, Nottingham, UK

OVERVIEW

- Teaching and learning evidence-based healthcare should be integrated into the rest of the healthcare curriculum rather than alongside it.
- Though knowledge of the five steps is important, students also need specifically to be taught how to apply evidence in practice.
- The evidence on which clinical practice is based should be made explicit.
- Students should be given opportunities to apply their knowledge of evidence-based healthcare to real-world problems.
- Shared decision-making and evidence-based healthcare should be taught together and not separately.
- Assessment should include the five steps, statistical concepts and application of skills to practice.

The learner's experience

Only a minority of healthcare professionals practise the five steps of evidence-based healthcare regularly in their professional practice (1). Healthcare professionals are expected to have skills for retrieving, appraising and integrating evidence. There is little information on how well professionals integrate evidence for decision-making into their daily practice. Although there are high, self-reported levels of interest in evidence-based medicine (EBM), barriers to its use by clinicians include lack of knowledge, skills and time (Box 10.1) (1). A majority of clinicians do consult clinical guidelines regularly. Since guidelines represent the synthesis of pre-appraised evidence into recommendations for clinical practice, this is encouraging. Differences in use across healthcare professions may reflect priority given to evidence-based healthcare across the various training programmes. However, interprofessional working and multidisciplinary care for patients suggest understanding evidence-based healthcare is important for all and should be addressed across all curricula. Given the fact that professionals appear to rely on others to produce resources which then become labelled 'evidence-based',

professionals need at least the skills to critically appraise key new evidence, particularly around specific, new or controversial recommendations (1).

Evidence is everywhere

Although there is a perception that evidence-based healthcare relates mainly to choice of diagnostic test or treatment intervention, there is also an evidence base for clinical assessment of the patient, that is, the history and examination. Students in all healthcare professions acquire and practice history taking and physical examination skills from an early stage of training. Despite the great advances in technology around clinical assessment, clinical assessment remains a very significant component in the formulation of both clinical reasoning, diagnosis and differential diagnosis (2–4). Advances in epidemiology and use of systematic reviews have improved the knowledge base of the history both at a population level and in its application to individuals (5). We understand better how symptoms are expressed individually and synergistically to produce disease. Though not well established for teaching purposes, research is increasing into symptom clusters, which may denote particular conditions or disease types (6). This evidence can be synthesised into resources to underpin the teaching of history taking in healthcare programmes (7). Similarly, models of evidence-based clinical communication facilitate the collection of clinical data from the patient history (8). Collaboration with patient actors (standardised patients) and patient volunteers within clinical skills teaching facilities enables this learning to occur in safe spaces for both patients and learners.

Evidence-based physical examination

Eliciting a physical sign is a diagnostic test. A sign is objective evidence of a patient's health found by physical examination. Signs may be normal and found in all patients. For example, the radial pulse and blood pressure are 'vital' signs as they are so important in denoting a patient's overall health in both acute and

ABC of Evidence-Based Healthcare, First Edition. Edited by John Frain.
© 2025 John Frain. Published 2025 by John Wiley & Sons Ltd.

Box 10.1 **Knowledge and use of evidence-based medicine in daily practice by health professionals**

Regular use of EBM in practice
• 14.2% used EBM regularly
• 15.6% used EBM occasionally
• 33.1% knew about EBM but did not use it
• 31.9% had just heard about EBM
• 4.0% do not know about EBM

Use of EBM-related sources
• 83.4% used clinical guidelines at least monthly
• 47.1% used PubMed
• 23.1% used the Cochrane Library
• 6.4% used other medical databases

Use by profession
• 12% of pharmacists use EBM
• 22% of nurses use EBM
• 36% of doctors use EBM

Source: Adapted from Lafuente-Lafuente et al. (1).

chronic illness. Evidence of change of the physical characteristics of the body caused by disease (e.g. clubbing of the fingers in respiratory disease) are also physical signs. Finding them is the purpose of physical examination. The presence of an established sign increases the probability of a patient having a particular condition or type of condition. The structure of a diagnostic accuracy study of a physical sign and the sources of bias are the same as any other diagnostic accuracy study (Figure 10.1). A reference test for the sign can be established, and the accuracy of the sign can be calculated using a 2 × 2 table. For example, in the assessment of a physical sign of anaemia, conjunctival pallor is the index test, and the laboratory haemoglobin level is the reference test. The resulting sensitivity and specificity can be used to calculate a likelihood ratio (LR) for the sign (Chapter 6), which is usable by the bedside (10).

Physical signs may be present or absent even when the patient does or does not have the target condition (false positive and false negatives). Teaching an evidence-based physical examination at the bedside facilitates discussion of sensitivity and specificity, validity, precision, reliability and similar concepts relevant to evidence-based healthcare. These discussions are grounded in the students' own experiences of eliciting the signs, making them explicit and more vivid. They are likely to be more readily retained and be transferrable to the understanding of evidence-based healthcare concepts more widely. Also relevant here are the concepts of intra- and inter-examiner variability and the kappa statistic (Table 10.1). These underline the operator dependence of all diagnostic tests. The value is expressed as kappa (k), where 0.0–0.2 is slight agreement, 0.21–0.40 is fair, 0.41–0.60 is moderate, 0.61–0.80 is substantial and 0.81–1.00 is perfect agreement (Table 10.1) (11). It may be appreciated that the individual kappa statistics for respiratory signs are low, suggesting subjectivity amongst examiners and the need for a consistent approach to the physical examination. Variation in the method of physical examination is a source of diagnostic error as well as anxiety amongst students as they approach summative assessments with worry about who will be examining them and their examiners' preferred method of physical examination. A further dimension to the discussion is that given the low kappa values of individual respiratory signs, the signs benefit from being used in combination. Of course, we can also provide students with evidence-based justification for the use of imaging, bronchoscopy and sputum culture to increase diagnostic accuracy whilst at the same time emphasising they also have limitations, and clinical judgement must always be exercised.

Table 10.1 Kappa values for the respiratory examination.

• Dullness to percussion	0.52
• Wheezes	0.43–0.93
• Chest expansion	0.38
• Bronchial breath sounds	0.32
• Crackles	0.30–0.63
• Cough	0.29
• Tachypnoea	0.25
• Breath sound intensity	0.23–0.46
• Tactile fremitus	0.01

Source: Adapted from Joshua et al. (11).

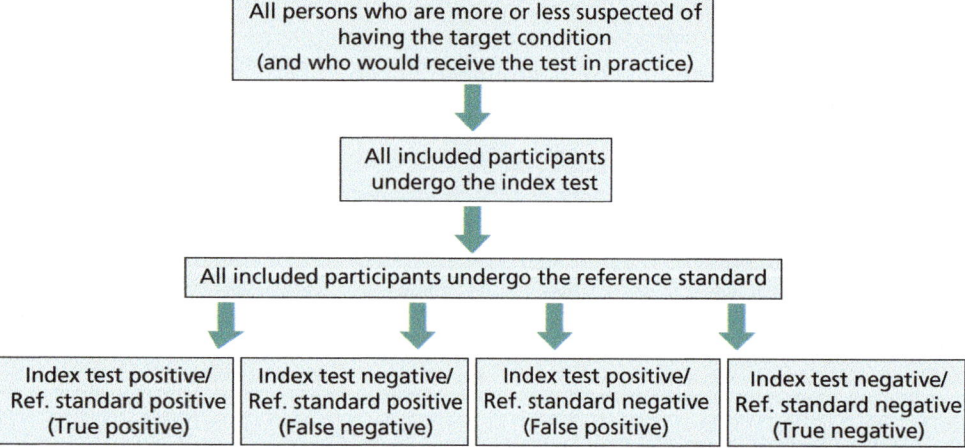

Figure 10.1 Flow chart outlining the structure of a diagnostic accuracy test. *Source:* Leeflang and Allerberger (9)/with permission of Elsevier.

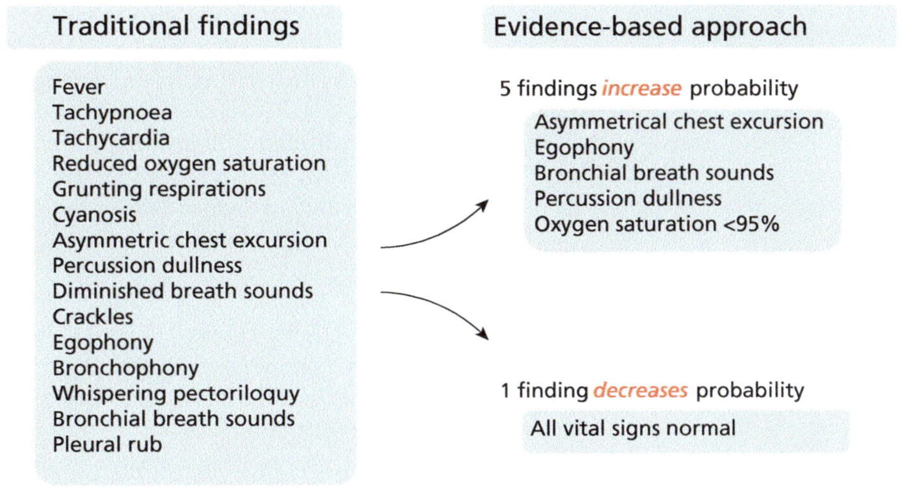

Traditional findings	Evidence-based approach
Fever Tachypnoea Tachycardia Reduced oxygen saturation Grunting respirations Cyanosis Asymmetric chest excursion Percussion dullness Diminished breath sounds Crackles Egophony Bronchophony Whispering pectoriloquy Bronchial breath sounds Pleural rub	**5 findings *increase* probability** Asymmetrical chest excursion Egophony Bronchial breath sounds Percussion dullness Oxygen saturation <95% **1 finding *decreases* probability** All vital signs normal

Figure 10.2 Diagnosis of lobar pneumonia. Textbooks present 15 traditional, physical findings of pneumonia (left), along with the assumption that each finding has similar diagnostic weight. The evidence-based method (right), based on the study of actual patients, shows that five findings accurately increase the probability of pneumonia and only one finding decreases it. *Source:* Cooper and Frain (12)/John Wiley & Sons.

Physical signs do have greater diagnostic accuracy when combined. Again, this can be taught to students as a component of bedside teaching and clinical reasoning (Figure 10.2). Doing so emphasises the importance of thorough clinical assessment and the increased likelihood of diagnostic error when history and examination are incomplete.

Clinical prediction rules

Where the evidence base for symptoms and signs can be established from diagnostic accuracy studies, clinical prediction rules have been developed. A prediction rule calculates the absolute risk of a condition or future outcome (13). Reliable rules should have been created using accepted methodological standards and frameworks. They should also have been evaluated and validated for use in the target population (13). A rule meeting these criteria has the potential for a positive impact on patient assessment. The scoring of the rule and thresholds for diagnosis can be established using Receiver Operating Characteristic (ROC) curves (Chapter 6). Context and derivation of the research on which the rule is based provide excellent opportunities for teaching critical appraisal. Many prediction rules are now available. Examples include the Wells score for deep venous thrombosis (DVT) and the TIMI score in acute myocardial infarction (MI). A comparison of the Centor and FeverPain scores in acute sore throat is shown in Table 10.2.

Tips for evidence-based bedside teaching

The principle that the history and physical examination should also be evidence-based is well established. The Rational Clinical Examination series has published a number of systematic reviews on both physical signs and conditions (15). Evidence summaries and textbooks of clinical examination have also been published (16, 17). In my own institution, our graduate entry students (GEMs) have been taught evidence-based clinical skills for almost 20 years. The development of such a course requires preparation of suitable

Table 10.2 Comparison of the Centor criteria and FeverPAIN clinical prediction score.

Centor criteria	FeverPAIN criteria
Tonsillar exudate Tender anterior cervical lymphadenopathy Fever greater than 38 °C Absence of cough	*Fever* during previous 24 hours *Purulence* (pharyngeal/tonsillar exudate) *Attend* rapidly (within three days after onset of symptoms) Severely *inflamed* tonsils *No* cough or coryza
Each item scores one point with maximum score of four A score of three or more has a sensitivity of 49%, a specificity of 82%, a positive LR of 2.68 and negative LR of 0.62 for streptococcal pharyngitis. A score of four has specificity of 95% (LR+ 3.85 and LR− 0.86)	Each item scores one point with maximum score of five A FeverPAIN score of 4 or more has low sensitivity (3.7%) but specificity of 98.1%

Source: Adapted from Seeley et al. (14), Frain (7).

teaching resources, including workbooks, films and faculty development. Box 10.2 summarises key tips for successful evidence-based bedside teaching (18).

Practising the five steps of evidence-based healthcare

Healthcare students commence their training enthusiastic about seeing patients, eliciting symptoms and signs and making diagnoses. Clinical skills training underpinned by the evidence for assessing the patients fosters an understanding of the nature of evidence and the need to question the basis for these skills in order to improve understanding and reasoning of diagnosis and management. This can be formalised into coursework in which their understanding of the five steps can be assessed. In the United Kingdom, the General Medical Council's *Outcomes for Graduates* stipulates the requirements of newly qualified doctors in understanding research (Box 10.3) (19).

Some students may meet these requirements through intercalated degrees, but the majority will not do so. Exposure to evidence should permeate training. Where training in evidence-based healthcare is abstract, didactic and not related to the student's own clinical experience and problem solving, the students quickly forget the skills they have learnt and may qualify without the requisite skills. This then carries forward into their future practice. Coursework based on the five steps will help achieve this. In my own institution, pre-clinical GEM students undertake coursework aligned to their first-year primary care placements in which they are asked to identify a patient in whom they have either performed or witnessed a particular clinical skill (Table 10.3). The chosen skill must be either an aspect of the patient's history, a clinical sign, a sequence of physical examination or a clinical prediction rule. This becomes the index test for an evaluation of the evidence for the skill. Framing of the assignment is based on three questions:

1 Was the chosen skill helpful in the management of the patient?
2 Is this skill one which can be recommended for use in similar patients more widely?
3 How could any gap in the existing evidence be addressed?

The assignment results in a 2000-word essay. Even for GEMs with previous experience of scientific research, the assignment results in an upskilling and enabling of the intended skills, which can be utilised further during clinical training.

The evidence-based healthcare curriculum

Supporting the aforementioned training still requires elements of workshop-based teaching, practice of skills and opportunities for feedback. These involve both research-based and clinical staff in a collaboration to ensure the knowledge base is established in students' minds. Knowledge and application can also be assessed through formats including single-best answer (SBA) assessments and Objective Structured Clinical Examination (OSCE) stations assessing shared decision-making and communication of risk (Box 10.4).

As discussed in Chapter 8, the principles of evidence-based healthcare, shared decision-making and communication of risk need to become more closely integrated, taught and practised together if individual clinicians are to more successfully practice evidence-based healthcare with patients.

Table 10.3 Course assignment and practice in the five steps of evidence-based healthcare.

Step	Action
Formulate a clinical question	• Identify a patient seen in practice • Obtain informed consent • Identify clinical skills relevant to the patient • Formulate a PICO question including a suitable reference test
Search for evidence	• Derive search terms from the PICO question • Define inclusion and exclusion criteria • Use the 6S pyramid to guide evidence retrieval from a range of medical databases using a 'top-down' approach
Appraise the evidence	• Select relevant evidence • Use a structured approach, including suitable appraisal tools • Evaluate the index and reference test, including statistical information
Apply to patient	• Reflect on the evidence – what was the validity and reliability of the chosen skill? Was it useful in the patient's management? • Can this skill be recommended for use more widely in clinical assessment of patients?
Evaluate the outcome	• What were the gaps in the evidence? • Is further research needed? • Formulate a further research question, including an outline methodology • Is an evidence base relevant to the history and examination more widely? • What are your reflections on your learning from undertaking this project?

Box 10.4 **Workshops to support training in the five steps of evidence-based healthcare**

- Introduction and philosophy of evidence-based healthcare
- Diagnosis and screening
- Briefing on the evidence base for a clinical skill coursework
- Search and retrieval skills
- Principles of study design
- Clinical trials
- Systematic reviews
- Statistical concepts
- Critical appraisal
- Qualitative research
- Health economics
- Shared decision-making
- Communicating risk to patients

Teaching strategies for evidence-based healthcare

The principle of understanding evidence and the magnitude of effects in research studies is relatively straightforward for students and teachers. The challenge for evidence-based healthcare training is facilitating its application to patients. Shared decision-making is now recognised as a key component of this (20). A scoping review

---

Box 10.5 **Recommendations for integration of shared decision-making and evidence-based healthcare**

- Make explicit the link between evidence-based healthcare and shared decision-making.
- Map the content of shared decision-making skills to the five steps of evidence-based healthcare with particular focus on step 4 'apply'.
- Provide simultaneous overview to learners of principles, steps and outcomes of shared decision-making and evidence-based healthcare.
- Include patients in programme development and delivery.
- Engage with students through multiple teaching and assessment strategies, including role modelling, patient actors, detailed and specific feedback and explanation or relevance.

Source: Adapted from Lehane et al. (21)/with permission of Elsevier.

---

of teaching strategies for shared decision-making found only a minority of 23 selected studies did so within the context of evidence-based healthcare (21). The most frequently cited barrier to shared decision-making is a lack of suitable training, knowledge and skills (22). Training programmes address the steps 'ask', 'acquire' and 'appraise' but rarely progress to 'apply' and 'addressing the outcome' (23). A key recommendation in addressing this is the avoidance of 'learning silos' typified by the teacher who says, 'Oh, we don't need to cover that, you'll do that somewhere else' (Box 10.5).

Support strategies include online, or perhaps AI-based, simulations (20). These provide the facility of detailed feedback on content and particularly the statistical nuances of accurate risk communication. Safe spaces help build confidence in skills with which clinicians clearly struggle. In Hoffman's study, the learner is required to answer four knowledge questions and perform three calculations (20). This cognitive load is commensurate with clinical practice when consulting with one patient. Online, or similar, practice will help to develop skills. However, face-to-face practice also needs to be provided. Learners can be guided with suggested forms of words (Box 10.6). Checklists or domains provide items for informal feedback and formative or summative feedback (Table 10.4).

Journal clubs

Journal clubs are common, popular and effective forums for practising critical appraisal for both students and qualified doctors. Again, these can be used to provide students with practice in the five steps, particularly if allied to clinical training and patient care. A US study evaluating the impact of a five-journal club course found increases in students' skills at formulating clinical questions, evidence retrieval and critical appraisal, though no change to students' overall knowledge of evidence-based healthcare (Figure 10.3) (24). Similar results were reported in a study among dental students in Pakistan (25). Journal clubs also form a valuable part of postgraduate training for maintaining and developing skills further (Box 10.7).

Box 10.6 **Suggested learner scripts for risk communication**

1 Assess preferences for communication
'Would you like me to go into more detail about the pros and cons of the treatment choices, including numbers and statistics'?
2 Explain the magnitude of risks using multiple frames
  ○ Both percentages and natural frequencies
'Based on who you are, medical experts estimate that your risk of developing colon cancer in your lifetime is 10%'.
'This is the same as saying that 10 people in 100 like you will develop colon cancer in their lifetimes'.
  ○ Both negative and positive frames
'Medical experts estimate that about 10 out of 100 people like you will develop colon cancer during their lifetimes'.
'You can also look at this in another way. 90 out of 100 people like you will stay free of colon cancer'.
  ○ Emphasise absolute risk reduction
'Studies show that taking DRUG X lowers people's risk of a heart attack by 25% or about one quarter. But to see if it is worth taking DRUG X, we need to count the number of people who are actually helped by DRUG X ...'.
'The studies show that DRUG X lowered the amount of people having heart attacks from 4 out of 100 to 3 out of 100. So, DRUG X helped about 1 person out of every 100 people who took it'.
3 Explain the meaning of the reference class
'One way to think about this is to imagine a group of 100 people like you, who have the following things in common (e.g. sex, age, family history of cancer, etc.). Of this group of 100 similar people, 10 will develop colon cancer in their lifetime'.
4 Acknowledge uncertainty
  ○ Meaning of chance/inability to predict single events
'We can't predict the future of any one person. Estimates of risk, of the chances, only tell us how many people in some group are likely to get cancer. They can't tell us who will get the disease or not'.
'Even if the risk of a complication from surgery is 10 out of 100, we don't know whether you will be one of the unlucky 10 who will suffer the complication, or the lucky 90 who will not'.
  ○ General scientific uncertainty
'Estimates of risk, of the chance of something happening, are not perfect because science is not perfect. We don't know everything we need to know to predict the future'.

Source: Han et al. (23)/with permission of Elsevier.

Table 10.4 Checklists for clinical communication and risk communication skills.

Risk communication process	Risk communication content
• Greeted patient appropriately and introduced self	• Discussed the quality, strength or weakness (e.g. validity, reliability and credibility) of the risk evidence
• Set the stage for discussion	• Specified the reference class (patient population) or to whom the risk estimates apply
• Assessed preferences for communication	• Specified the time period over which the risk estimates apply
• Checked understanding and elicited questions	• Explained the magnitude of risk using both negative and positive frames
• Gave information clearly using plain language and avoided jargon	• Explained risk estimates using both proportions (e.g. 9 out of 100) and percentages (e.g. 9%)
• Demonstrated responsiveness, empathy, respect and professionalism	• Discussed differences between baseline risk and modified risk in absolute terms (absolute risk reduction) or both absolute and relative terms
• Elicited patient concern and responded appropriately	• Acknowledged general uncertainty in all risk estimates using qualitative terms
• Gave a well-paced explanation	• Acknowledged uncertainty due to chance or randomness (inability to predict single events)
• Maintained a dialogue	• Placed the magnitude of risks in context by comparing to risks of other outcomes (e.g. other diseases, treatments and familiar events)
• Demonstrated empathy	
• Actively listened	
• Built a therapeutic relationship throughout the consultation	
• Closed consultation appropriately	

Source: Han et al. (23)/with permission of Elsevier.

Learner attitudes

Students are generally positive about evidence-based care. They enjoy opportunities to practise skills and apply them whilst on clinical placements. It is seen as relevant to their current training and to their future practice (26). Perceived barriers to their learning include poor role modelling of skills by their clinical teachers and constraints on time and resources in a busy curriculum (26). Students who were taught the five steps report more frequent use of journal literature searches during clinical training. A study of student's use of appropriate databases for clinical questions during placement found 51% using one source, 42% using two and 6% using three. These tended to be point-of-care resources and PubMed (27). Positive student experiences are associated with application of the skills, completing a research-based project, active engagement in the learning and opportunities to integrate the research concepts with clinical practice (28). The diverse range of student research interests can be challenging for tutors (28).

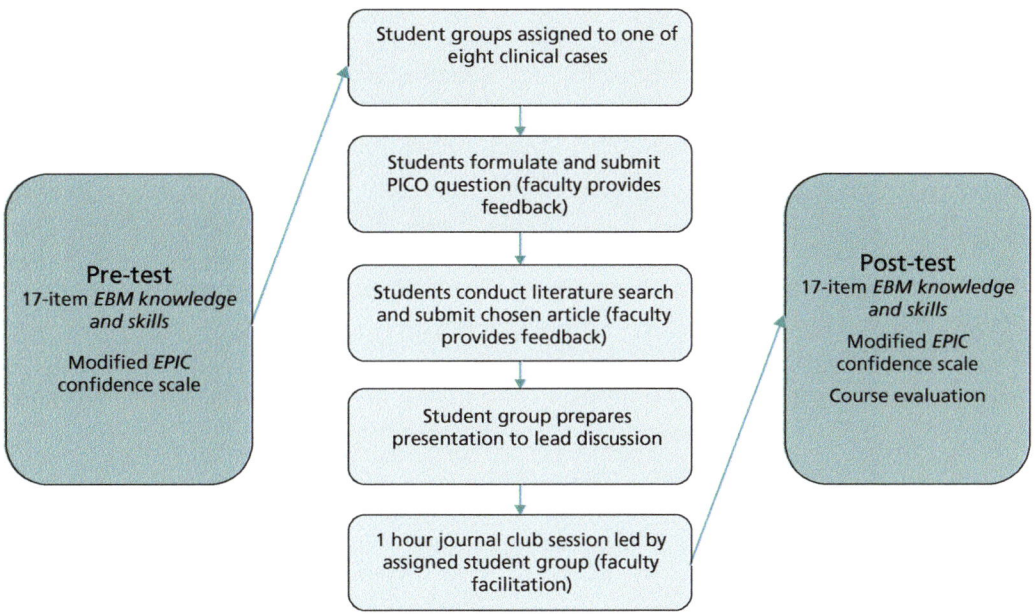

Figure 10.3 Flow chart for evaluation of the effectiveness of a journal club for improving evidence based medicine skills in preclinical medical students. *Source:* Cahill et al. (24)/Springer Nature.

Box 10.7 **Teaching application of evidence-based healthcare at postgraduate level**

There is evidence that even experienced clinicians struggle to apply EBM in practice, so how can this be taught in postgraduate training?

In postgraduate speciality training in general practice in the United Kingdom, there are specific challenges. Over 60% of the specialist trainees (STs), in some areas, are International Medical Graduates (IMGs). Firstly, establishing what training in areas such as EBM and shared decision-making (SDM) all the STs have had is important. At times there are significant cultural differences, meaning SDM is not as common in healthcare. We concentrate on communication skills and culturally important aspects of the consultation as the STs start their three years of speciality training.

Statistics are a significant part of the applied knowledge test (AKT) examination which relies on the doctors seeing many patients and applying their knowledge. STs are fully aware of the importance of understanding and applying statistics, so this is a case of assessment driving learning.

In our programme, we have a journal club encouraging the STs to learn to read and critically appraise the literature. In general, they do not look at systematic reviews but are used to using clinical guidelines. They also learn to use clinical decision tools, such as risks of breast cancer with HRT or taking anticoagulation in atrial fibrillation.

Practising having conversations with patients which communicate risk, more practical application of statistics and use of decision aids can help to ensure shared decision-making is done well and doctors feel confident to do this.

Dr Anna Frain,
Programme Director for Derby Specialist Training Programme for General Practice, Derby, UK

Summary

In this chapter, we have outlined the need to support students in translating evidence into practice. Their training needs to provide them with opportunities to apply evidence according to where they are in their development. Healthcare students in all disciplines will see patients and learn to assess them through history, examination and procedures. An evidence base exists for these skills as well as a teaching methodology. Clinical assessment can be used as a starting point for students to apply evidence in their own practice. Allied to suitable teaching, assignments and assessment, they can use these opportunities to build their confidence and skills in evidence-based healthcare. Crucial to this also are opportunities for deliberate practice and detailed, specific feedback in shared decision-making and the communication of risk to both simulated and real patients.

References

1 Lafuente-Lafuente, C., Leitao, C., Kilani, I. et al. (2019). Knowledge and use of evidence-based medicine in daily practice by health professionals: a cross-sectional survey. *BMJ Open* 9 (3): e025224. https://doi.org/10.1136/bmjopen-2018-025224. PMID: 30928940; PMCID: PMC6475442.

2 Peterson, M.C., Holbrook, J.H., Von Hales, D. et al. (1992). Contributions of the history, physical examination, and laboratory investigation in making medical diagnoses. *West J Med* 156 (2): 163–165.

3 Martina, B., Bucheli, B., Stotz, M. et al. (1997). First clinical judgment by primary care physicians distinguishes well between nonorganic and organic causes of abdominal or chest pain. *J Gen Intern Med* 12 (8): 459–465.

4 Rudwaleit, M., Metter, A., Listing, J. et al. (2006). Inflammatory back pain in ankylosing spondylitis: a reassessment of the clinical history for application as classification and diagnostic criteria. *Arthritis Rheum* 54 (2): 569–578.

5 Rasmussen, S., Søndergaard, J., Larsen, P.V. et al. (2014). The danish symptom cohort: questionnaire and feasibility in the nationwide study on symptom experience and healthcare-seeking among 100 000 individuals. *Int J Family Med* 2014: 187280.

6 Fei, F., Siegert, R.J., Zhang, X. et al. (2023). Symptom clusters, associated factors and health-related quality of life in patients with chronic obstructive pulmonary disease: a structural equation modelling analysis. *J Clin Nurs* 32 (1–2): 298–310.

7 Frain, J. (2025). *Exploring Symptoms: An Evidence-based Approach to the History*. Oxford: Wiley.

8 Silverman, J.K.S. and Draper, J. (2013). *Skills for Communicating with Patients*, 3e. Oxford: Radcliffe.

9 Leeflang, M.M.G. and Allerberger, F. (2019). How to: evaluate a diagnostic test. *Clin Microbiol Infect* 25 (1): 54–59. https://doi.org/10.1016/j.cmi.2018.06.011. Epub 2018 Jun 12. PMID: 29906592.

10 McGee, S. (2002). Simplifying likelihood ratios. *J Gen Intern Med* 17 (8): 646–649. https://doi.org/10.1046/j.1525-1497.2002.10750.x. PMID: 12213147; PMCID: PMC1495095.

11 Joshua, A.M., Celermajer, D.S., and Stockler, M.R. (2005). Beauty is in the eye of the examiner: reaching agreement about physical signs and their value. *Intern Med J* 35: 178–187.

12 Cooper, N. and Frain, J. (2023). *ABC of Clinical Reasoning*, 2e. Oxford: Wiley.

13 Cowley, L.E., Farewell, D.M., Maguire, S., and Kemp, A.M. (2019). Methodological standards for the development and evaluation of clinical prediction rules: a review of the literature. *Diagn Progn Res* 22 (3): 16. https://doi.org/10.1186/s41512-019-0060-y. PMID: 31463368; PMCID: PMC6704664.

14 Seeley, A., Fanshawe, T., Voysey, M. et al. (2021). Diagnostic accuracy of Fever-PAIN and Centor criteria for bacterial throat infection in adults with sore throat: a secondary analysis of a randomised controlled trial. *BJGP Open* 5 (6). https://doi.org/10.3399/BJGPO.2021.0122.

15 JAMANetwork (2024). The rational clinical examination. https://jamanetwork.com/collections/6257/the-rational-clinical-examination (accessed 28 August 2024).

16 Talley, N.J. and O'Connor, S. (2021). *Clinical Examination: A Systematic Guide to Physical Diagnosis*, 9e. Sydney: Elsevier Churchill Livingstone.

17 McGee, S. (2021). *Evidence-based Physical Diagnosis*, 5e. St Louis, MO: Saunders Elsevier.

18 Mookherjee, S., Hunt, S., and Chou, C.L. (2015). Twelve tips for teaching evidence-based physical examination. *Med Teach* 37 (6): 543–550. https://doi.org/10.3109/0142159X.2014.959908. Epub 2014 Oct 1. PMID: 25270026.

19 General Medical Council (2020). *Outcomes for Graduates*. London: GMC.

20 Hoffmann, T.C., Légaré, F., Simmons, M.B. et al. (2014). Shared decision making: what do clinicians need to know and why should they bother? *Med J Aust* 201 (1): 35–39. https://doi.org/10.5694/mja14.00002. PMID: 24999896.

21 Lehane, E., Curtin, C., and Corrigan, M. (2023). Teaching strategies for shared decision-making within the context of evidence-based healthcare practice: a scoping review. *Patient Educ Couns* 109: 107630. https://doi.org/10.1016/j.pec.2023.107630. Epub 2023 Jan 13. PMID: 36689886.

22 Waddell, A., Lennox, A., Spassova, G., and Bragge, P. (2021). Barriers and facilitators to shared decision-making in hospitals from policy to practice: a systematic review. *Implement Sci* 16 (1): 74. https://doi.org/10.1186/s13012-021-01142-y. PMID: 34332601; PMCID: PMC8325317.

23 Han, P.K., Joekes, K., Elwyn, G. et al. (2014). Development and evaluation of a risk communication curriculum for medical students. *Patient Educ Couns* 94 (1): 43–49. https://doi.org/10.1016/j.pec.2013.09.009. Epub 2013 Sep 19. PMID: 24128795.

24 Cahill, E.M., Ferreira, G., and Glendinning, D. (2023). The effectiveness of a journal club for improving evidence-based medicine skills and confidence in pre-clerkship medical students. *Med Sci Educ* 33 (2): 531–538. https://doi.org/10.1007/s40670-023-01779-y. PMID: 37251208; PMCID: PMC10061358.

25 Mumtaz, S. and Sabir, S. (2022). Evaluating critical appraisal skills by introducing journal clubs to preclinical dental students using the assessing competency in evidence-based medicine (ACE) tool through pre and post-testing. *Cureus* 14 (11): e31535. https://doi.org/10.7759/cureus.31535. PMID: 36532935; PMCID: PMC9754061.

26 Ilic, D. and Forbes, K. (2010). Undergraduate medical student perceptions and use of evidence based medicine: a qualitative study. *BMC Med Educ* 19 (10): 58. https://doi.org/10.1186/1472-6920-10-58. PMID: 20718992; PMCID: PMC2931522.

27 Nicholson, J., Kalet, A., van der Vleuten, C., and de Bruin, A. (2020). Understanding medical student evidence-based medicine information seeking in an authentic clinical simulation. *J Med Libr Assoc* 108 (2): 219–228. https://doi.org/10.5195/jmla.2020.875. Epub 2020 Apr 1. PMID: 32256233; PMCID: PMC7069825.

28 Ferri, D., Moore, C., and Mun, K.J. (2023). Student and educator perceptions of an evidence-based medicine research curriculum: recommendations for research curriculum development. *Uni Toronto Med J* 100. https://doi-org.nottingham.idm.oclc.org/10.33137/utmj.v100i1.38689 (accessed 28 August 2024).

Glossary

Absolute risk reduction   the proportion of patients who are spared the adverse outcome due to having received the intervention rather than being in the control group.

Adverse event   an event which occurs when a patient has been provided with healthcare or participated in a research study.

Adverse reaction   these include medication side effects, injury, psychological harm, trauma or death resulting from healthcare or participation in healthcare research. They may be preventable or unpreventable, foreseen or unforeseen.

Alternative hypothesis   the opposite of a null hypothesis, the alternative proposes there is a statistically significant relationship between two variables.

Applied research   research undertaken with the intention of improving patient care and outcomes, the delivery of healthcare and the effectiveness of healthcare staff.

Artificial intelligence   technology enabling computers and machines to simulate human learning, problem solving and understanding.

Association   exploring association between variables establishes the strength and direction of any relationships between the variables and enables comparison between groups.

Bias   in research, bias occurs when systematic error occurs in the sampling or conduct of a study such that one outcome or answer is encouraged over others.

Blinding   information having the potential to influence study results is withheld from one or more groups of participants in the study.

Causation   the reason or cause for the disease process, injury or study outcome.

Chief investigator   the person who takes overall responsibility for the design, conduct and reporting of a study.

Clinical prediction rule   a tool which uses the presence of symptoms and signs of a condition to estimate the probability of a disease or health outcome.

Clinical questions   these are questions about aetiology or causation, diagnosis, therapy, prognosis and economic. They may be either background or foreground questions.

Comparison of groups   this is the comparison of two participant groups in a study, usually one receiving an intervention and the other a control. The mean values for variables in each group enable comparison of two groups or conditions to assess whether they are significantly different or not.

Concealment   ensuring the random allocation of participants to intervention or control groups occurs without knowledge of which patient will receive which treatment.

Confidence interval   in statistics, the probability of a particular population parameter will fall between two set values.

Confounding variable   an unmeasured third variable which may affect the relationship of the cause and effect between two variables being studied in a clinical trial or research project.

Correlation   a measure which expresses the linear relationship between two variables – they change together at a constant rate.

ABC of Evidence-Based Healthcare, First Edition. Edited by John Frain.
© 2025 John Frain. Published 2025 by John Wiley & Sons Ltd.

Database	a structured, organised collection of information (data) stored electronically in a computer system.	Health economics	related to issues of efficiency, effectiveness, value and behaviour in the production, delivery and consumption of healthcare.
Decision analysis	the philosophy, methodology and professional values necessary to understand and address how decisions are made and evaluated.	Heterogeneity	the quality or state of consisting of dissimilar or diverse elements.
Diagnosis	identification of a disease, condition or injury from its symptoms, signs and results of investigations.	Homogeneity	in a systematic review, this is a measure of similarity between selected studies.
Diagnostic accuracy study	a cross-sectional or cohort study in which at least one diagnostic test is compared with a reference test to estimate its diagnostic accuracy.	Hypothesis	a proposed explanation made on the basis of limited evidence as a starting point for further investigation or experimentation. Usually expressed as a null or alternative hypothesis.
Diagnostic test	a test used to confirm if a person has a particular condition or disease based on their symptoms and signs.	Impact factor	it is used as a proxy-level metric of the importance of a journal.
Effectiveness	the degree of beneficial effect occurring from an intervention in 'real-world' conditions.	Implementation science	the scientific study of methods to promote the systematic uptake of research findings into clinical practice.
Efficacy	whether an intervention produces the expected results in ideal conditions.	Incidence	the rate of new cases or events over a specified time period in a population at risk of the event.
Endpoint	a measurable event or outcome which can help determine if an intervention being studied is beneficial.	Inclusion	the practice or policy of providing equal access to opportunities and resources for people who might otherwise be excluded or marginalised, such as those who have physical or mental disabilities and members of other minority groups.
Event rate	the number of events (including multiple events per person) divided by the total person – years of experience.		
Evidence synthesis	combining evidence from a range of sources to inform debates and issues on specific issues.	Index test	the procedure, test or physical sign that is being evaluated in a diagnostic accuracy study.
Face validity	the degree to which a test, procedure or assessment appears effective in terms of its stated aims.	Informed consent	permission granted in full knowledge of the possible consequences – usually the risks and benefits of medical care.
Fixed effects model	a statistical model which assumes each unit has its own fixed effect rather than a random probability or effect.	Intention to treat analysis	a measure to include in an analysis of all randomised patients, regardless of adherence to the study protocol, treatment or lack of treatment received or their withdrawal from the study.
Forrest plot	a graphical representation which summarises data from multiple studies in a single image.		
Funnel plot	a graphical scatter plot used to check for existence of publication bias in studies of evidence synthesis such as systematic reviews.	Iterative	building, refining and improving a project.
Grey literature	materials and research produced outside of traditional and academic publishing, including reports, policy documents and academic theses.	Kappa	a calculation corrected for the effect of chance which assesses inter-rate agreement.
		Large language model	machine learning models which can understand and generate human language tasks.
Hazard ratio	how often an adverse event occurs in one group compared to another; a hazard ratio of greater than 1 implies increased risk and less than 1 implies a smaller risk.	Machine learning	computer systems which are able to learn and adapt without explicit instructions but rather based on algorithms and statistical models.

Mechanistic reasoning	an inference from underlying mechanisms of how an intervention produced a study outcome.	Randomisation	the process of selecting or ordering things in a random way to reduce bias and interference by irrelevant factors.
Null hypothesis	the claim that the effect being observed in a study does not exist.	Raw data	data which has not yet been processed, coded, formatted or analysed.
Number needed to treat	the number of patients needing to be treated to avoid one additional adverse outcome (e.g. death).	Reference test	the best available method for establishing whether a medical condition is present or not.
Odds ratio	a measure of association between an exposure and an outcome.	Relative risk	the probability of an event occurring in an exposed group versus the event occurring in an unexposed group, usually expressed as a ratio.
Open label	a research study in which there is no complete blinding and where participants and researchers may be aware of the assigned intervention.	Representation in research	addressing the historical failure to include underserved groups on the basis of gender identity, ethnicity and sexual orientation.
Paradigm	a standard, perspective or set of ideas.	Risk	the possibility of an adverse event.
Patient and public engagement	ensuring the outcomes of research are disseminated to patients and the public.	Sampling	the selection of individuals from within a population of interest. It may be randomised or non-randomised.
Patient and public involvement	patients and the public with relevant experience contribute to how research is designed, conducted and disseminated.	Shared decision-making	a collaborative process between a patient and a health professional to reach a decision about healthcare.
Post-marketing surveillance	activity undertaken by manufacturers to monitor drugs after they reach market following clinical trials.	Study sponsor	a person, organisation or group which funds and oversees a research study.
Power	the probability a study will detect a predetermined level of difference in measurement between two groups.	Subgroup analysis	dividing the study participants into groups for the purpose of making comparisons between them.
Prevalence	the proportion of a population affected by a particular medical condition.	Symptom cluster	a group of two or more symptoms related to one another and occurring together.
Principal investigator	the researcher who leads the research team.	Systematic literature review	the identification, selection and critical appraisal of research literature to answer a pre-formulated question.
Prognosis	the likely outcome or course of a disease; the chance of recovery or recurrence.	User-led research	research directed or led by service users, for example, patients.
Proof of concept	a demonstration of work in determining whether an idea can be turned into reality.	Validity	how accurately a study method measures what it was designed to measure. Validity may be internal or external.
Publication bias	the outcome of a study influences the decision whether or not to publish it.	Variable	a person, place, biological factor or phenomenon which a study is trying to measure. A dependent variable is the outcome of interest, such as a disease, while an independent variable will affect the dependent variable.
Random effects model	variations in outcomes which cannot be explained by the observed variables.		

Bibliography

Biddle, K., Blundell, A., and Sofat, N. (2023). *Understanding Clinical Research: An Introduction*. Banbury: Scion Publishing Ltd.

Crombie, I.K. (2021). *Evidence in Medicine: The Common Flaws, Why they Occur and How to Prevent Them*. Oxford: Wiley.

Goodfellow, J.A. (2012). *Understanding Medical Research: The Studies That Shaped Medicine*. Oxford: Wiley-Blackwell.

Greenhalgh, T. (2017). *How to Implement Evidence-based Healthcare*. Oxford: Wiley-Blackwell.

Harris, M., Taylor, G., and Jackson, D. (2024). *Clinical Evidence Made Easy: The Basics of Evidence-based Medicine*, 2e. Banbury: Scion.

Hochman, M.E. and Hochman, S.D. (2022). *50 Studies Every Doctor Should Know: The Key Studies that Form the Foundation of Evidence-based Medicine*. Oxford: Oxford University Press.

Howick, J. (2011). *The Philosophy of Evidence-based Medicine*. Oxford: Wiley.

Jolley, J. (2020). *Introducing Research and Evidence-based Practice for Nursing and Healthcare Professionals*, 3e. Routledge.

Knotterus, J.A. and Buntinx, F. (2011). *The Evidence Base of Clinical Diagnosis: Theory and Methods of Diagnostic Research*. Oxford: Wiley-Blackwell.

Linsley, P. and Kane, R. (2022). *Evidence-based Practice for Nurses and Allied Health Professionals*, 5e. Thousand Oaks, CA: Sage.

Offredy, M. and Vickers, P. (2010). *Developing a Healthcare Research Proposal: An Interactive Student Guide*. Oxford: Wiley-Blackwell.

Straus, S.E., Glaziou, P., Richardson, W.S., and Haynes, R.B. (2019). *Evidence-based Medicine: How to Practice and Teach EBM*, 5e. Elsevier.

The Multi-Regional Clinical Trials Center (2021). *The MRCT Center of Brigham and Women's Hospital and Harvard. Achieving Diversity, Inclusion and Equity in Clinical Research: Guidance Document and Supplementary Toolkit*. Cambridge, MA: MRCT Center.

Zipkin, D.A. (2023). *Teaching Evidence-based Medicine*. Cham, Switzerland: Springer.

Systematic reviews

Deeks, J.J., Bossuyt, P.M., Leeflang, M.M., and Takwoingi, Y. (2023). *Cochrane Handbook for Systematic Reviews of Diagnostic Test Accuracy (Wiley Cochrane Series)*. Oxford: Wiley-Blackwell.

Higgins, J.P.T., Thomas, J., Chandler, J. et al. (2019). *Cochrane Handbook for Systematic Reviews of Interventions (Wiley Cochrane Series)*, 2e. Oxford: Wiley-Blackwell.

Khan, K.S. and Zamora, J. (2023). *Systematic Reviews to Support Evidence-based Medicine: How to Appraise, Conduct and Publish Reviews*. Abingdon, OX: CRC Press.

Critical appraisal

Gosall, N. and Gosall, G. (2015). *The Doctor's Guide to Critical Appraisal*, 4e. Knutsford: Pastest.

Greenhalgh, T. (2019). *How to Read a Paper: The Basics of Evidence-based Medicine and Healthcare*, 6e. Oxford: Wiley.

Qualitative research

Cresswell, J.W. (2024). *Qualitative Inquiry and Research Design: Choosing Among Five Approaches*, 5e. Thousand Oaks, CA: Sage.

Cresswell, J.W. and Cresswell, J.D. (2023). *Research Design – International Student Edition: Qualitative, Quantitative and Mixed Method Approaches*, 6e. Thousand Oaks, CA: Sage.

Smith, J.A., Flowers, P., and Larkin, M. (2021). *Interpretative Phenomenological Analysis: Theory, Method and Research*, 2e. Thousand Oaks, CA: Sage.

Statistics

Grove, S.K. and Cipher, D.J. (2024). *Statistics for Nursing Research*, 4e. Elsevier.

Hossain, M. (2021). *Making Sense of Medical Statistics: A Bite Sized Visual Guide*. Cambridge: Cambridge University Press.

Kirkwood, B.R. and Sterne, J.A.C. (2025). *Essential Medical Statistics*, 3e. Oxford: Wiley-Blackwell.

Salkind, N.J. and Frey, B.B. (2019). *Statistics for People Who (Think They) Hate Statistics*, 7e. Thousand Oaks, CA: Sage.

Scott, I. and Maazhindu, D. (2014). *Statistics for Health Care Professionals: An Introduction*, 2e. London: Sage.

Useful Tools and Websites

General

BMJ Best Practice
https://bestpractice.bmj.com/info/

Centre for Evidence Based Medicine – Oxford, UK
https://www.cebm.net

Cochrane Collaboration
https://www.cochrane.org

Declaration of Helsinki
https://www.wma.net/wp-content/uploads/2016/11/DoH-Oct2008.pdf

EBM Tools
https://bestpractice.bmj.com/info/us/toolkit/ebm-tools/

Evidence-Based Medicine
https://fhshrwelcome.mcmaster.ca/did_you_know/evidence-based-medicine/

Evidence-Based Medicine Toolbox
https://ebm-tools.knowledgetranslation.net

Good Clinical Practice (GCP)
https://www.nihr.ac.uk/health-and-care-professionals/training/good-clinical-practice.htm

James Lind Library
https://www.jameslindlibrary.org

Joanna Briggs Institute (JBI)
https://jbi.global

National Institute for Health and Care Research
https://www.nihr.ac.uk

Nuremburg Code
https://ori.hhs.gov/content/chapter-3-The-Protection-of-Human-Subjects-nuremberg-code-directives-human-experimentation

UK Policy Framework for Health and Social Care Research
https://www.hra.nhs.uk/planning-and-improving-research/policies-standards-legislation/uk-policy-framework-health-social-care-research/

Search and retrieval skills

Databases
AMED
https://www.ebsco.com/products/research-databases/allied-and-complementary-medicine-database-amed

CINAHL
https://www.ebsco.com/products/research-databases/cinahl-database

Cochrane Library
https://www.cochranelibrary.com

Embase
https://www.embase.com/landing?status=grey

Medline
https://www.nlm.nih.gov/medline/medline_overview.html

Psychinfo
https://www.apa.org/pubs/databases/psycinfo

PubMed
https://pubmed.ncbi.nlm.nih.gov

Searching skills
Paperpile
https://paperpile.com/g/search-online-research-database/
https://paperpile.com/g/systematic-literature-review/

PRISMA statement
https://www.prisma-statement.org/

ABC of Evidence-Based Healthcare, First Edition. Edited by John Frain.
© 2025 John Frain. Published 2025 by John Wiley & Sons Ltd.

Principles of study design

The EQUATOR Network
https://www.equator-network.org

HRA Decision Tool
https://www.hra-decisiontools.org.uk/ethics/EngresultN1.html

PROSPERO
https://www.crd.york.ac.uk/PROSPERO/

Research Design Service London
https://www.rds-london.nihr.ac.uk

Trial registries
https://clinicaltrials.gov
https://www.isrctn.com
https://eudract.ema.europa.eu

Statistical concepts

MedCalc
https://www.medcalc.org/index.php

Stata
https://www.stata.com

Statistics at Square One, 9th Edition
https://www.bmj.com/about-bmj/resources-readers/publications/statistics-square-one

Critical appraisal

Cochrane Risk of Bias Tool
https://methods.cochrane.org/bias/resources/rob-2-revised-cochrane-risk-bias-tool-randomized-trials

Critical Appraisal Skills Programme (CASP)
https://casp-uk.net

ETQS tool for Qualitative Studies
https://phdliteraturereviews.pbworks.com/f/Evaluation+Tool+for+Qualitative+Studies.pdf

GRADE recommendations
https://www.gradeworkinggroup.org

International Committee of Medical Journal Editors guidelines
https://www.google.com/search?client=safari&rls=en&q=international+committee+of+medical+journal+editors+(icmje)+guidelines&ie=UTF-8&oe=UTF-8

QUADAS-2
https://www.bristol.ac.uk/population-health-sciences/projects/quadas/quadas-2/

Evidence into practice

MAGIC: Shared decision making
https://www.health.org.uk/funding-and-partnerships/programme/magic-shared-decision-making

Option grids
https://www.ebsco.com/sites/g/files/nabnos191/files/acquiadam-assets/Option-Grid-Take-Away-Guide.pdf

Wiser Choices
https://www.wiserhealthcare.org.au/category/decision-aids/

Teaching and learning evidence-based healthcare

Directory of Open Access Journals
https://doaj.org

Rational Clinical Examination
https://jamanetwork.com/collections/6257/the-rational-clinical-examination

Index

ABC of Evidence-Based Healthcare, First Edition. Edited by John Frain.
© 2025 John Frain. Published 2025 by John Wiley & Sons Ltd.